She Does KETO

D0523935

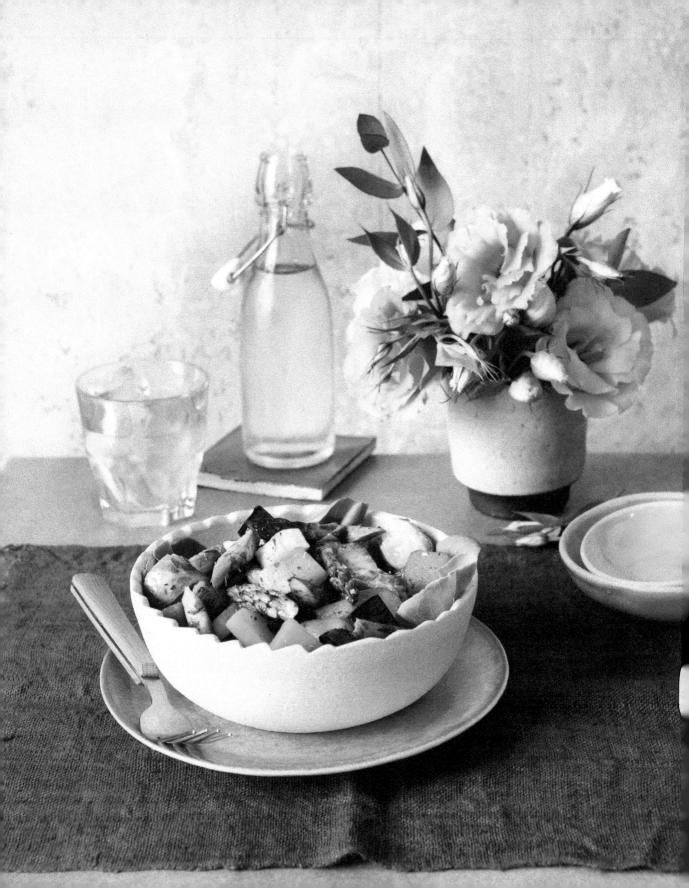

She Does
KETO

THE COMPLETE KETOGENIC DIET FOR WOMEN

GIGI ASHWORTH

PHOTOGRAPHY BY NADINE GREEFF

ROCKRIDGE
PRESS

Copyright © 2019 by Rockridge Press, Emeryville, California

No part of this publication may be reproduced, stored in a retrieval system, or transmitted in any form or by any means, electronic, mechanical, photocopying, recording, scanning, or otherwise, except as permitted under Sections 107 or 108 of the 1976 United States Copyright Act, without the prior written permission of the Publisher. Requests to the Publisher for permission should be addressed to the Permissions Department, Rockridge Press, 6005 Shellmound Street, Suite 175, Emeryville CA 94608.

Limit of Liability/Disclaimer of Warranty: The Publisher and the author make no representations or warranties with respect to the accuracy or completeness of the contents of this work and specifically disclaim all warranties, including without limitation warranties of fitness for a particular purpose. No warranty may be created or extended by sales or promotional materials. The advice and strategies contained herein may not be suitable for every situation. This work is sold with the understanding that the Publisher is not engaged in rendering medical, legal, or other professional advice or services. If professional assistance is required, the services of a competent professional person should be sought. Neither the Publisher nor the author shall be liable for damages arising herefrom. The fact that an individual, organization, or website is referred to in this work as a citation and/or potential source of further information does not mean that the author or the Publisher endorses the information the individual, organization, or website may provide or recommendations they/it may make. Further, readers should be aware that Internet websites listed in this work may have changed or disappeared between when this work was written and when it is read.

For general information on our other products and services or to obtain technical support, please contact our Customer Care Department within the U.S. at (866) 744-2665, or outside the U.S. at (510) 253-0500.

Rockridge Press publishes its books in a variety of electronic and print formats. Some content that appears in print may not be available in electronic books, and vice versa.

TRADEMARKS: Rockridge Press and the Rockridge Press logo are trademarks or registered trademarks of Callisto Media Inc. and/or its affiliates, in the United States and other countries, and may not be used without written permission. All other trademarks are the property of their respective owners. Rockridge Press is not associated with any product or vendor mentioned in this book.

Interior and Cover Designer: Emma Hall
Photo Art Director: Karen Beard
Editor: Pippa White
Production Editor: Erum Khan

Photography © 2019 Nadine Greeff. Author photo courtesy of Adam Sheridan.

ISBN: Print 978-1-64152-357-8 | eBook 978-1-64152-358-5

TO MY FATHER,
who has no problem sharing a can of anchovies
or tomato paste with me.

TO MY MOTHER,
who lets me eat her salmon sashimi and sometimes
seared albacore sashimi, as well.

TO MY SISTER,
who loves crispy salmon skin and eel just as much as I do.

TO MY BROTHER,
who always shares photos of his delicious meals with me,
but not the actual meals.

TO MY HUSBAND,
who only once took food off my plate without asking,
and survived to tell the tale.

AND TO MY NEWBORN SON,
Truman, who is currently screaming because he wants food.

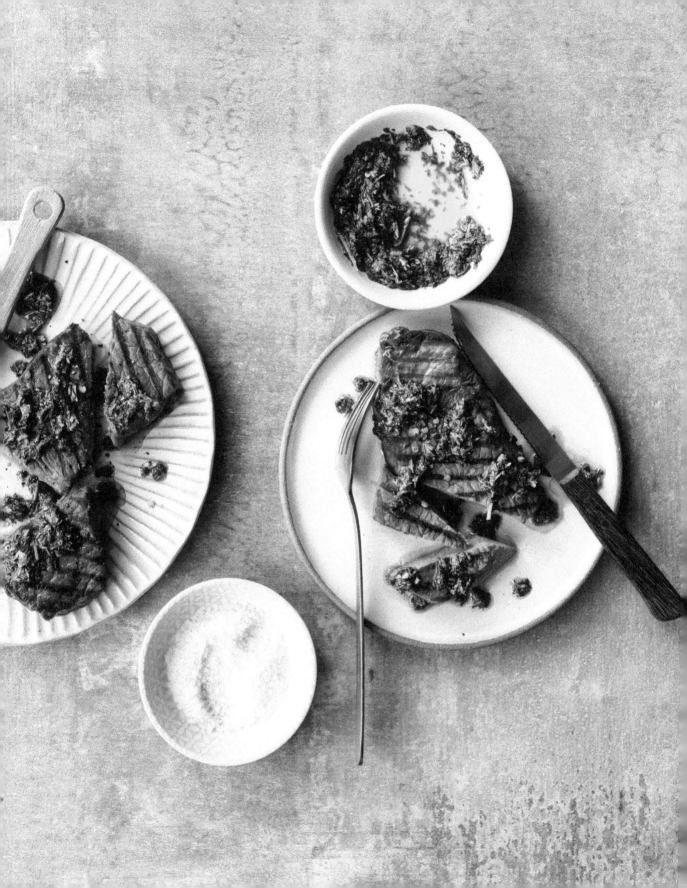

Contents

Introduction ix

PART I: MAKE KETO WORK FOR YOU 1

1 Keto for Women 3

2 Setting Yourself Up for Success 17

The 21-Day Meal Plan 27

PART II: RECIPES 45

3 Breakfast 47

4 Sides & Snacks 63

5 Soups & Salads 79

6 Vegetarian Main Dishes 99

7 Seafood & Poultry 117

8 Beef & Pork 147

9 Desserts 179

10 Beverages 195

11 Sauces & Dressings 207

Measurement Conversions 219

References 220

Recipe Index 221

Index 223

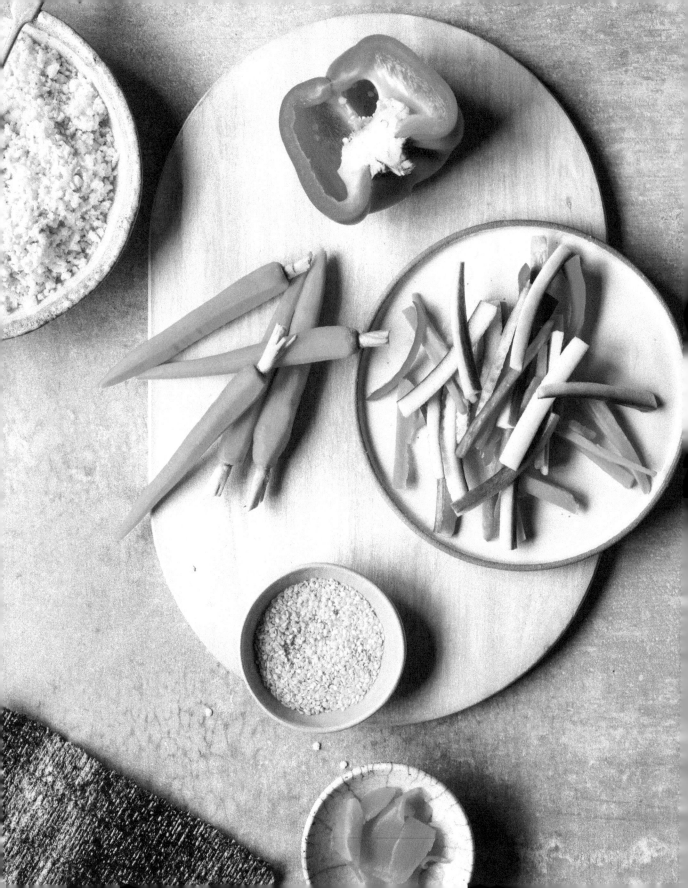

Introduction

If you opened up 13-year-old GiGi's closet door and rummaged through her crumpled-up clothing on the floor, you'd most likely find an open box of Brown Sugar Cinnamon Pop-Tarts®. Those frosted toaster pastries were one of the many food items my mother strictly forbade, yet I somehow still managed to snag a box of them every month or so. If those treats weren't available, I'd dive into my brother's secret stash of Chewy Chips Ahoy! cookies. If I was in a salty mood—and, let's be honest, I could be quite salty as a teenager—I'd ask my sister if she would share her Triscuits.

Now, if you opened up present-day GiGi's closet door, you'd find lots of workout clothing and no food. If you opened up my pantry, you'd see none of the items I used to slyly enjoy when no one was watching. Instead you'd find healthy snacks like roasted seaweed, low-sodium and sugar-free jerky, raw veggies, and lots of cans of sardines and salmon. I'd like to say that the transition to this new diet was due to my maturing as a person. It was not.

While I was at boarding school in high school, I began competitively snowboarding, which made me pay attention to my physical self in a new way. I started to notice how frequently I didn't feel well after eating, but I couldn't figure out what was causing my gastric distress. After some time, I was diagnosed with the sexy-sounding *cecal volvulus*, a condition that can obstruct digestion, and which led to the removal of my large intestine. At the same time, I was diagnosed with food intolerances and an autoimmune disease.

After that, my mother, a doctor, recommended *her* way of eating; she had been practicing a diet remarkably similar to the modern-day ketogenic diet for quite some time. She sent me a book, and in the margins she had written little notes highlighting the most important take-away: Eat a diet high in fat with a good amount of protein and little to no carbohydrates.

That's right: no carbohydrates. For an athlete, eating a low-carbohydrate diet sounded ridiculous. It was pretty much unheard of back in 2002.

During the transition from cookie monster to meatball monster (yep, I subsisted mostly on meatballs when I was in boarding school), I did my best to consume only low-carbohydrate or what we'd now call keto-approved foods. In the early phases of experimenting, I learned that gluten, sugar, and fruit were off the table for me. My body just couldn't process them, confirming the way forward. (I also discovered that some keto-approved foods don't work for me, including nuts, dairy, and soy. For this reason, you won't see many recipes in this book that focus on those ingredients, though I have included some, because your body may be different from mine!)

Despite the hurdles, I was able to make the keto lifestyle work for me, and my body began to heal. After years of eating this way, I feel the best I ever have. My personal journey with food and doing research to understand my body was the driving force behind my earning a journalism degree from the University of Colorado at Boulder and a graduate certificate from the Tufts University Friedman School of Nutrition Science and Policy.

Today, the keto diet is becoming increasingly popular, especially among women, which is why I wanted to write this book. My nutrition education and longtime experience with the diet has made me well-versed in its effects on a woman's body. Going keto has made a huge difference in my life, helping me fuel my athletic pursuits and even regulate my menstrual cycle. I hope it will make a positive impact in your life, as well!

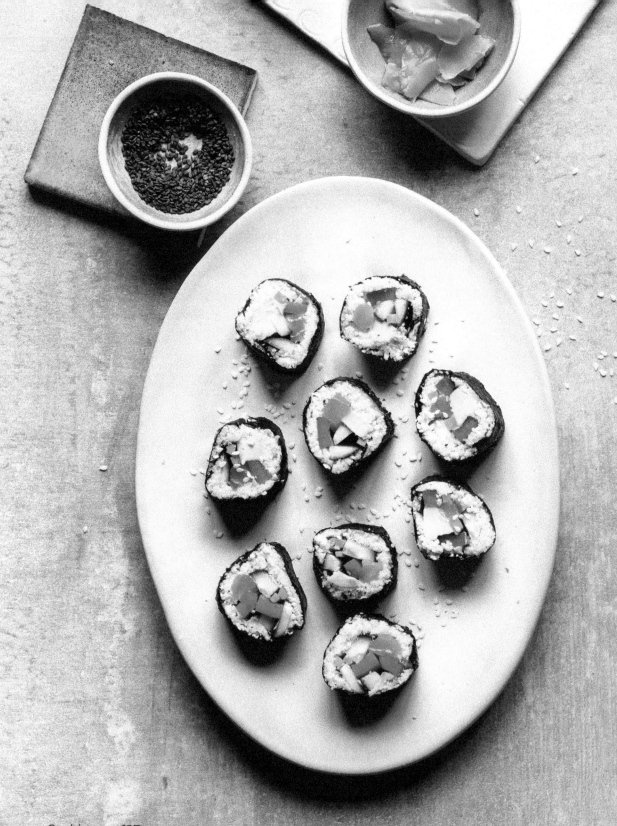

Sushi, page 127

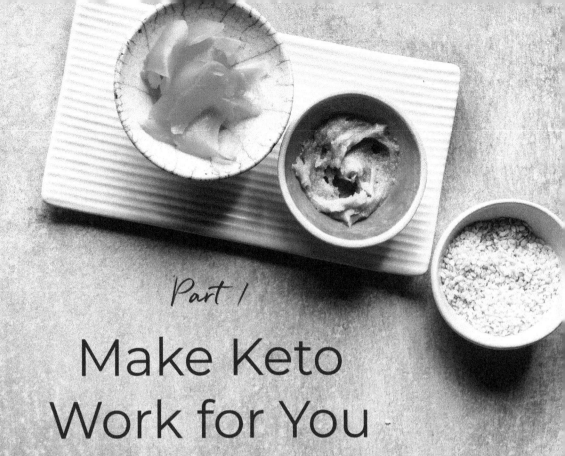

Part 1

Make Keto Work for You

Ladies, it's time to break the rules! That's right, this book goes against the general dietary recommendations advocated in the United States. You've most likely been told for your entire life that you should eat a diet heavy on carbohydrates and light on fats. While this advice is still being pushed by the USDA, there have been many studies concluding that this way of eating is not as wholesome as once thought. The evidence is piling up that a diet high in (healthy) fats and lower in carbohydrates, i.e., the keto diet, will improve your health! So put down that slice of bread slathered in lite margarine and pick up that crispy piece of bacon dunked in guacamole! Breaking the rules has never tasted so good!

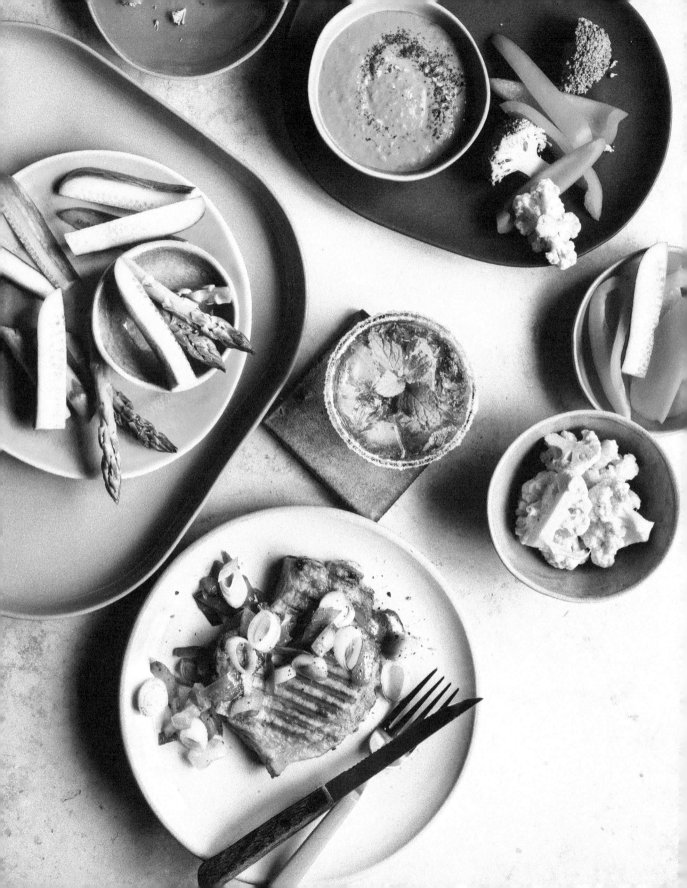

Chapter 1

Keto for Women

While following the ketogenic diet is ultimately easy, convenient, and delicious, a little education is absolutely necessary in order to make it that way. This chapter's job is to cover the basic principles and science behind the keto diet as well as the ways it uniquely affects women.

How the Term "Woman" Is Used in This Book

For the purpose of this book, we are going to use the terms "woman" and "female" interchangeably. In many cases where the book explores the physiology of women, you will notice that we focus on cisgender women. This is not intended to exclude or alienate anyone, and the great news is that the recipes in this book will work for anyone because keto is good for everyone, even if the science is a bit different from what's laid out in this chapter.

Why Keto?

The first thing to know about this diet is that technically you will lose fat the same way you would on any other diet. All diet plans work by taking more fat out of cells than what gets put into them. There's a catch, though. If you are not reducing carbohydrate intake, the only way to do this is to trick your body into thinking it's starving by eating drastically less than you normally do, which is not a good idea—especially for women.

Women's bodies are more complex than men's due to their finely tuned hormones. Women's bodies detect caloric deficits and nutritional shortages more quickly and suffer the consequences more rapidly. The beauty of the keto diet is that due to simple carbohydrate restriction, women can experience fat loss without severely restricting calories and micronutrients. Focusing on nutrient-dense whole foods and avoiding nutrient-poor foods is the key to being successful on the keto diet.

The Nutritional Needs of Women

It's probably not news to you that women have a unique physiology and thus have different nutritional needs from men. First and foremost, our calorie needs are different. Men generally have larger bodies, greater muscle mass, and a need for more calories. Even a man with the same height and weight as his female counterpart will burn roughly 400 more calories per day than she will. Lucky us, right?

Beyond that, it has been well established that we need more vitamins and minerals due to hormonal changes, menstruation, and childbearing. The most important of these vitamins and minerals include calcium, vitamin D, a vitamin B complex, iron, iodine, and magnesium. These are notoriously difficult to obtain in adequate amounts on a calorie-restricted diet. Thankfully the keto diet is no such thing, which is why it's better for your body.

Here are some of the vitamins and minerals that are plentiful on the keto diet.

CALCIUM Women are more susceptible to osteoporosis than men, which increases the risk of fractures. Foods rich in calcium that are keto staples include full-fat dairy products, sardines, salmon, and kale.

VITAMIN D From helping the body absorb calcium and building stronger bones to decreasing inflammation, vitamin D has been dubbed a miracle cure by many. While the best way to get it is by going outside and soaking up those sunrays, you can also eat plenty of fatty fish, egg yolks, mushrooms, and animal liver—all foods that are emphasized on the keto diet!

B VITAMINS The entire B complex includes B1, B2, B3, B5, B6, B9, B12, and biotin, which are water-soluble essential nutrients. When you think of B9, also known as folate, think green. High-folate foods include spinach, collard greens, mustard greens, asparagus, broccoli, and avocado. B12 is generally found naturally in animal products, including fish, meat, poultry, eggs, and milk.

IRON This mineral helps with red blood cell formation, wound healing, immune function, and energy production. Women are often iron-deficient due to blood loss during their menstrual cycles. Iron can be found in keto-friendly foods such as red meats, liver, and poultry.

IODINE This mineral is crucial for healthy fetus development during pregnancy. Keto-approved foods that are high in iodine include seafood, seaweed, eggs, and iodized salt.

MAGNESIUM This is a mineral that affects more than 300 enzyme systems in a woman's body and regulates biochemical reactions, including protein synthesis, nerve regeneration, blood sugar control, and blood pressure regulation. Foods that contain a lot of magnesium include all leafy greens and avocado.

As you can see, the keto diet contains foods with essential nutrients specific to the needs of a woman's body, so you don't need to worry about creating a vitamin or mineral deficiency by eating this way.

Why Starting a New Diet Can Be Hard

Changing the way you eat is hard. In the beginning of any diet, you have to override cravings for things your body has grown to expect you will eat.

The keto diet is a regimen that may initially feel even more challenging because it flies in the face of so many nutritional dicta you've probably been taught since grade school. Although the diet has gained in popularity, there are many critics who will try to dissuade you from even starting. The best advice I can give you is to do your own research. Knowing how and why this diet works is just as important as knowing what to eat.

One of the most common mistakes women make when starting the keto diet is not eating enough calories from fat. Eating healthy fat will send signals to your body that there is an abundance of food available. This message means your body will not dive into metabolic conservation mode as it does when there is a caloric deficit. Eating healthy fat also gives you a psychological boost. Being able to eat rich foods and actually feel satisfied rather than starving yourself on low-calorie, air-filled rice cakes is a gift, as far as I'm concerned. This satisfaction will motivate you to stay on this diet and reap all of its benefits.

How the Ketogenic Diet Works

As you're aware, fuel is necessary to power us through everything from sleeping to exercise, and we get this fuel from food. But you may not be aware that there are two sources of this fuel: We can get it from glucose (from carbohydrates) or from fatty acids (from fats). The fuel your body uses is mostly determined by the composition of your diet. When eating a high-carbohydrate diet (you know, full of processed flours, breads, pasta, whole grains, root veggies, and tropical fruits—aka the standard American diet), your body will break this food down into simple sugars called glucose.

In both men and women, glucose is the default fuel. When eating carbohydrates, especially in their refined form such as breads and pasta, your insulin rapidly increases. This allows glucose to be taken up by your muscles and brain for energy. Any excess glucose is then stored as glycogen in your liver. Roughly 6 to 24 hours after a meal, your insulin levels fall, and the glycogen stored in your liver releases glucose to keep blood sugar levels steady. Several hours later, if you still have not eaten, gluconeogenesis, the breakdown of protein, occurs to provide some energy. Now, if you still have not eaten for one or two days, or you have taken in minimal sugar, your body starts searching for another fuel source: fat. The process of breaking down fat for fuel is called ketosis.

What Is Ketosis?

Ketosis is a normal process that our bodies undergo. Even if you're not trying to reach ketosis, you may very well have experienced a mild form of it if you ever have skipped a meal or exercised for more than an hour, or simply did not eat carbohydrates one day. Whenever your energy needs increase and there aren't enough incoming carbohydrates, your body adjusts by using fat without any health detriment. This compensation is a natural part of life from an evolutionary point of view. Our bodies have evolved to deal with food scarcity. The keto diet works by naturally changing your metabolism to your advantage.

What Are Macros? Why Are They Important?

In contrast to micronutrients (such as vitamins and minerals), which we need in small amounts to survive, macronutrients (aka macros) are substances that are essential in relatively large amounts. There are only three macros: carbohydrates, protein, and fat. Finding the right balance to get into and stay in ketosis is critical.

The breakdown of macronutrients you should strive for daily on the keto diet is as follows:

70% TO 75% FAT

15% TO 20% PROTEIN

5% TO 15% CARBS

The exact amount of carbohydrates that must be restricted for ketosis to occur differs among individuals. Exercise, stress, sleep, genetics, and even the types of carbohydrates and fats we eat also figure into the equation. Everybody is unique, so the amount of carbohydrates Sue over there is eating may be too much or too little for you.

On the keto diet you will need to eat enough protein to preserve your lean body mass and provide satiety. Protein is absolutely essential for tissue repair, immune function, and making hormones and enzymes. General guidelines vary significantly, but to avoid muscle loss make sure not to go below the daily recommendation (.36 grams per pound of body weight per day).

Last but not least, we all need adequate amounts of fat for energy, absorbing certain vitamins, providing protective cushions for organs, and maintaining cell membranes. If you are limiting carbohydrates and eating the right amount of protein to preserve muscle, the rest of your dietary requirements will be met by fat. As a matter of fact, fats are the majority of the calories you consume on this diet. Does this mean you should be eating bacon all day every day? Not exactly. While bacon is allowed, it's important to eat healthy fats. In the next chapter, we'll go over exactly which foods to eat and which to avoid on the keto diet.

What Happens to My Body on Keto?

To summarize all this info, if you restrict eating sugars and carbohydrates, your body will run low on glucose and will have to reach into its fat cells to start burning fat for energy. In this situation, your body begins to run on a special kind of fat called ketones, which are actually the brain's preferred energy source. Ketones provide you with renewed mental clarity, and they have also been found to be more efficient than glucose as a fuel for your cells.

Knowing When to Eat: Intermittent Fasting

In the past, dietitians have recommended three meals a day with up to three snacks between to increase metabolism and prevent hunger. Recent research suggests that the opposite is healthier: eating less frequently, commonly called fasting.

Many people combine keto with intermittent fasting to get through a plateau in their efforts to lose weight. Once you obtain ketosis, fasting becomes easier, and the fat you burn comes from your own stores, not simply the extra fat you are eating.

The key to healthy fasting is making sure you are controlling *when* you eat, rather than just not eating at all. Many people confuse fasting with starving. Fasting is about manipulating *the timing* of your calorie intake. Some fasting plans call for calorie reduction, and it's important for women to ensure that they are getting enough nutrients, so if you are planning to fast, please do so responsibly.

There are a few methods of IF, so you can audition one style at a time and see which works best for your lifestyle, though intermittent fasting is not required for keto.

THE LEANGAINS APPROACH (16/8 METHOD): Fast for 16 hours and eat only within an eight-hour window, say 10 a.m. through 6 p.m.

THE 5:2 REGIMEN: Eat only 500 to 600 calories for two days per week. The rest of the week eat your normal calorie allotment.

THE EAT-STOP-EAT PLAN: Fast for 24 hours, once or twice a week.

ALTERNATE-DAY FASTING: Fast for 24 hours, then eat your normal amount for the next 24 hours, then you fast again, and so forth.

THE WARRIOR DIET: Popularized by fitness expert Ori Hofmekler, this diet promotes eating very minimally during the day and then chowing down on a feast during a four-hour eating window.

SPONTANEOUS MEAL SKIPPING: If you don't feel like eating a meal, then skip it. If you don't feel like eating the next meal, skip it. If you do feel like eating your following meal, you can.

The Benefits of Keto

While your goal may be to lose weight, there's a slew of benefits for your body on keto.

Wellness

WEIGHT LOSS People used to believe that eating fat would cause it to go directly to their fat cells and that sugar would simply be used as energy. That has been proven wrong. Sugar stimulates insulin, and gets transformed into fats without you ever having eaten a trace of fat! Now, if you simply eat fat (and no sugar), it will not stimulate insulin, so your blood sugar will remain stable. At the same time, since fat is more energy-stable than sugar, it can provide your body with lots of energy for a much longer time. It will no longer require you to eat every two hours. You will automatically eat less, resulting in effortless weight loss. Although calories still count, the way to decrease them is the opposite of what you and I were taught in school.

INCREASED ENERGY Who doesn't want and need more energy? After being on a keto diet for three weeks, most women report an increase in energy accompanied by a lack of craving for carbohydrates, though the exact timing may differ. One of the main reasons for this increased energy is that once your body has adjusted to using a new fuel (ketones), the ketone molecules produce more biochemical energy than glucose, so your body works more efficiently. This will give you more stable energy rather than highs followed by energy crashes.

MENTAL CLARITY Often, women on a keto diet report feeling an increased alertness and focus. Researchers believe these results are most likely due to ketones providing an alternate fuel source and altering brain chemistry as well as stabilizing insulin, all of which translates to improved mental clarity. Numerous studies have shown improvements in epileptic patients as well as enhanced cognitive ability in some people with Alzheimer's disease.

BETTER SLEEP Some women report sleep problems when they first start the ketogenic diet, but interestingly, many go on to report better sleep once their bodies are used to the diet. One fascinating area of research points to a brain chemical called adenosine. Adenosine increases during the day, gradually promoting sleep. Studies show that the keto diet promotes adenosine activity in the body, helping to relax the nervous system and thus potentially improving sleep.

CLEARER SKIN The most exciting recent discovery is that the keto diet is anti-inflammatory and could help remedy many conditions for us ladies, including acne. When you reduce inflammation, changes can be seen immediately in your skin, with less redness and fewer breakouts. This also has tremendous implications for arthritis, psoriasis, eczema, irritable bowel syndrome (IBS), and other diseases involving inflammation and pain.

More research needs to be done in all of these areas, but studies are beginning to confirm what many women have intuitively felt were the beneficial effects of the keto diet.

Health

There are many health conditions that either uniquely affect women or affect women more frequently than men. The keto diet has been shown to help with several of them, which we'll briefly explore here.

POLYCYSTIC OVARY SYNDROME (PCOS)

One of the most common endocrine disorders in women is polycystic ovary syndrome (PCOS), said to be caused by hormone imbalance. According to Medscape, roughly 4 to 12 percent of women have PCOS but many don't even know it. Symptoms include excessive hair growth, irregular periods, difficulty getting pregnant, and high blood sugar. Scientists still do not know exactly what causes PCOS, but the accepted theory is that it results from a combination of genetics and lifestyle. A 2005 study found that when obese women with PCOS were placed on a keto diet for 24 days, their body weights decreased by 17 percent, testosterone levels lowered by 22 percent, and fasting insulin levels saw a 54 percent decrease. In 2017, another study showed that the keto diet reduced circulating insulin levels, which improved hormonal imbalances and resumed ovulation, resulting in improved pregnancy rates.

ENDOMETRIOSIS AND UTERINE FIBROIDS

You've probably heard of endometriosis, even if you have no idea what it is. It is yet another condition that affects women, and it occurs when the uterine lining, normally found inside of your uterus, grows outside of your uterus. According to Medscape, it occurs in about 6 percent to 10 percent of women in the United States. Symptoms of endometriosis include abdominal pain, heavy periods, and infertility. Although doctors have not identified a cause, genetics may play a role. Some theories suggest endometriosis might be an autoimmune condition or could be related to high estrogen levels. The same is true of uterine fibroids. Many physicians believe that an environment of high insulin and estrogen in a woman's body may contribute to fibroid growth as well as endometriosis, so, again, the lower insulin levels achieved on a keto diet could help.

AUTOIMMUNE CONDITIONS

Autoimmune conditions are more prevalent in women than in men by a factor of two to one. There are 80—yes, 80—autoimmune conditions that result in your immune system mistakenly attacking either a part of your body, like your skin or joints, or your whole body, as with lupus. Autoimmune conditions and diseases have been on the rise over the past couple of decades, and some scientists believe that high sugar and highly processed foods increase inflammation, which might set off autoimmune responses. According to Jeff Volek, PhD, RD, the chief science officer at Virta Health, the keto diet has been shown to decrease inflammation and could help in the treatment of autoimmune conditions. These benefits are still being researched so if you have an autoimmune condition, ask your doctor's opinion about going keto.

THYROID CONDITIONS

Oh, guess what?! Women are *also* more likely than men to experience thyroid dysfunction. Luckily the keto diet can be beneficial for thyroid conditions. When done correctly, eating keto stabilizes blood sugar levels, which allows for a balanced production of thyroid hormones. This is much better for your body than the roller-coaster effect that the typical American diet has on blood sugar.

Keto and the Female Body

Fat Metabolism and Hormones

Let me just say this loud and clear: Women's bodies process fat differently from men's bodies. When women and men consume more carbohydrates than they burn, extra calories are converted to fat by a complex mechanism and stored in the body as fat. This is where the similarities stop. In menstruating women, a continual rise in glucose and insulin can disrupt ovulation. Without ovulation, progesterone cannot be produced, sending women into a state of high estrogen, also known as estrogen dominance. The irony is that once the fat cells form from too many carbohydrates, the cells themselves will begin secreting estrogen, which is also a fat-storing hormone like insulin. The key to keeping this cruel cycle from getting out of control is to focus on preventing insulin levels from rising in the first place, rather than on decreasing estrogen or forcing ovulation by taking pills. One of the easiest ways to do this is through the keto diet and the delicious recipes found in this book.

Cortisol

Cortisol, also known as the stress hormone, helps boost your energy so you can take on the day. But many of us get too stressed out and our cortisol spikes, which has all sorts of effects on our bodies, including insomnia. Once your body has adjusted to eating keto and has built up enough enzymes to process fat as fuel, your cortisol levels will balance out naturally, leaving you calm, yet energetic—the perfect combo!

Tips for Getting the Most Out of Your Keto Diet

The ketogenic diet has many benefits for women, but it has to be done correctly.

QUALITY Women need to eat high-quality, nutrient-dense foods like eggs, avocados, fatty fish, nuts, olives, and high-fat, free-range meat and cheese. Eating bacon and pork rinds can get you into ketosis, but eating salmon with asparagus drizzled with olive oil will get you healthy. Eating real whole foods rather than processed bars and shakes is also a must for cellular health and regulating hormones.

CALORIES When starting the keto diet, women need to eat extra fats to regulate the fat-burning machinery in their cells. By increasing fat intake, you tell your body that there is no calorie deficit and an abundance of food. As you become more fat-adapted, you will use your own fat tissue and can decrease dietary fat. If you find yourself not losing weight after a month or so, consider tracking calories to see how many you are actually eating.

CARBOHYDRATES When it comes to carbohydrates, stay away from processed foods made with refined starches and added sugars, but don't skimp on vegetables. You can eat quite a lot of healthy vegetables to supply yourself with necessary minerals and vitamins without going overboard on carbohydrates.

PROTEIN Finding the perfect amount of protein depends on your weight and activity level. Too much protein can take you out of ketosis, but it's rare for women to eat too much protein. When possible, protein should be divided up throughout the day because your body can only use so much at a time for muscle synthesis.

FATS The biggest hurdle with fat is giving yourself permission to eat it. The next hurdle is figuring out the right kinds to eat. You can spend your days eating low-carb junk foods, or you can eat sardines on a bed of lettuce. While both will get you into ketosis, only one will make you healthy.

Since a majority of your calories will come from fat on the keto diet, it is absolutely crucial that you eat good fats, including olives, extra-virgin olive oil, avocados and avocado oil, almonds, Brazil nuts, macadamia nuts, pecans, pumpkin seeds, coconut oil, and butter.

EXERCISE Pairing keto with exercise is great, but be kind to yourself when beginning the diet; go easy on high-intensity exercise at first. Ketosis is a simple tool to help you achieve better health, but don't let it stress you out.

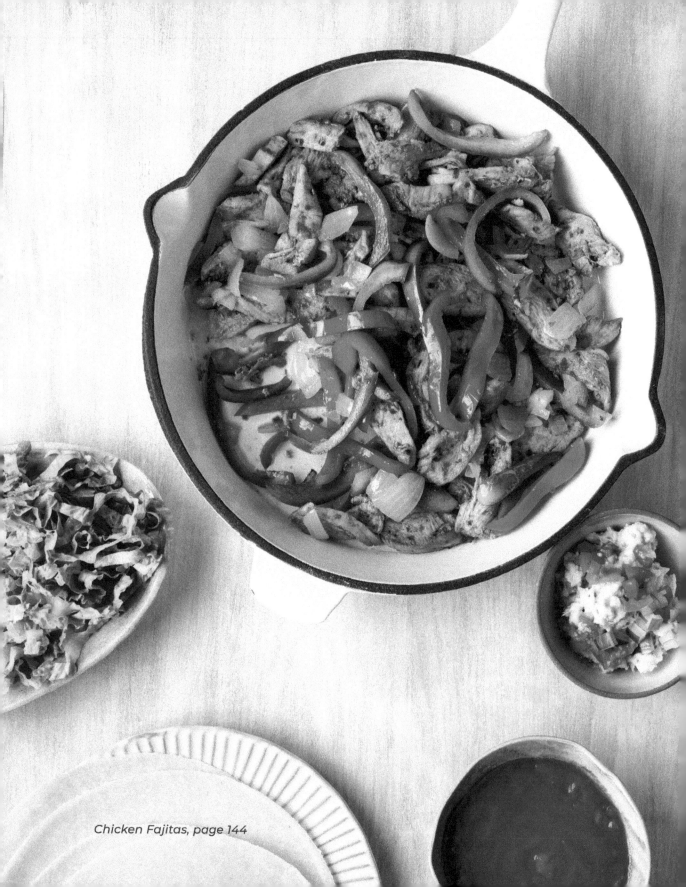

Chicken Fajitas, page 144

Chapter 2

Setting Yourself Up for Success

I am beyond thrilled that you're still here! As a thank-you for sticking around, get ready to start drooling, because we are talking food. We are going to dive into the foods that are keto stars (as well as name those that are not). On top of that, I will discuss the importance of planning ahead, so you don't go rabid hyena on a few dozen doughnuts when hunger pangs hit.

Know What to Eat

Generally, it's a good idea to opt for nutrient-dense foods, as mentioned in chapter 1. That means devouring pumpkin sprinkled with cinnamon and erythritol (a sweetener that has no effect on blood sugar) as opposed to a highly processed cinnamon bun.

Foods to Embrace

FATS

Animal Fats	Nut Butters	Quality Oils	Other
· Butter	· Almond butter	· Avocado oil	· Avocado
· Ghee	· Cocoa butter	· Coconut oil	· Coconut milk, full-fat
· Lard	· Coconut butter	· Extra-virgin olive oil	· Nuts (almonds, pecans, macadamia nuts, walnuts)
· Mayonnaise		· Macadamia oil	
· Tallow		· MCT oil	· Olives

PROTEIN

Beef	Organ Meats	Seafood	Steak
· Ground	· Collagen powder	· Salmon	· Filet
· Tenderloin	· Liver	· Sardines	· Flank
Chicken	· Tripe	· Scallops	· Rib eye
· Breast	Pork	· Sea bass	· Skirt
· Ground	· Bacon	· Shrimp	Turkey
· Quarters	· Chops	· Trout	· Ground
· Thighs	· Ground	· Tuna	· Quarters
· Whole	· Sausage		· Slices, precooked
Eggs	· Tenderloin		· Thighs
			· Whole

VEGETABLES

Artichokes	Cauliflower	Endive	Lettuce
Asparagus	Celery	Fennel	Mushrooms
Bok choy	Chard	Garlic	Okra
Broccoli	Chives	Green beans	Onions
Brussels sprouts	Cucumber	Kale	Peppers
Cabbage	Eggplant	Leeks	Radicchio

Radishes	Spinach	Tomatoes	Zucchini
Rhubarb	Sprouts	Water chestnuts	

FLAVORINGS

Black pepper, freshly ground	Fresh herbs (basil, cilantro, mint, oregano, parsley, rosemary, thyme, etc.)	Lemon	Vinegars (apple cider, balsamic, and red wine)
Dried herbs and spices		Lime	
		Mustard (yellow/Dijon)	
		Pink Himalayan salt	

BEVERAGES

Bone broth	Seltzer/ sparkling water, unflavored	Tea (unsweetened and not instant)	Water
Coffee (unsweetened)			

Foods to Eat in Moderation

Dairy (1 cup max per day)

- Cheese, full-fat
- Cream, heavy
- Greek yogurt, full-fat, plain

Fruits (1 cup max per day)

- Blackberries
- Blueberries
- Raspberries
- Strawberries

Foods to Avoid

- Most fruits: apples, bananas, oranges, etc. (Fruit has sugar in the form of fructose, which contributes to additional carbs and can't be processed by the body, so it is stored as fat.)
- Starchy vegetables: potatoes, sweet potatoes, plantains, butternut squash, etc.
- All grains and starches: bread, wheat, corn, rice, cereal, etc.
- Beer, cider, and sweet wines/liquors
- Refined oils: vegetable, grapeseed, canola, soybean, and corn
- Margarine

- Sugar of all kinds: white and brown sugars, honey, maple syrup, agave, high-fructose corn syrup, and evaporated cane juice
- Artificial sweeteners: Splenda, Sweet'N Low, Equal, Truvia, etc.
- Processed foods
- Soda/diet soda
- Fruit juice
- Fruit-based smoothies
- Energy drinks
- Low-fat and diet products (including sugar-free foods)

Planning Your Macros

It's important to understand the macronutrient balance when it comes to eating keto, or else you may never reach ketosis.

As discussed in chapter 1, macronutrients are fats, carbohydrates, and protein. We need these nutrients to, well, keep us alive. Healthy fat should take up roughly 70 percent to 75 percent of your diet, while carbohydrates should range anywhere from 5 percent to 15 percent of your diet. Round this out with a moderate amount of protein, 15 percent to 20 percent, and you're eating the keto way.

An ideal keto meal for someone trying to maintain their weight would include 6 to 8 ounces of roast salmon with a cup of broccoli that's been cooked in avocado oil or another healthy oil. If you're trying to lose weight on the keto diet, the same meal using a 4- to 6-ounce piece of salmon with less fat would work. Macronutrient ratios are extremely important to keep you satiated, but when it comes to weight loss, it's about calories in versus calories out.

You may be thinking, "This sounds great, but how on earth can I calculate my macronutrients?" There are a lot of macronutrient calculators online. All you have to do is plug in your personal information (such as age, height, weight, activity level, and what your goals are) and—*bam*—your results will be presented to you.

After living the keto lifestyle for such a long time, I no longer plan or count my macronutrients. It's become second nature to me, and hopefully it will become so to you.

Prepping Your Meals

Raise your hand if you've seen meal-planning photos on Instagram. Well, since I can't actually see you raising your hand, I am going to describe the #mealprepsundays photos that abound these days. Basically, people have 7 to 10 containers filled with protein, fat, and carbohydrates, parceled out for the week. You may have scoffed at such planning in the past, but since you are already trying a new diet, why not try something that will

The Keto Flu

Some people give up on the keto diet after just a few days due to feeling "lousy." Typical complaints include fatigue, light-headedness, brain fog, headaches, nausea, insomnia, dizziness, irritability, and/or upset stomach. This is sometimes called the keto flu, despite the fact that it is not an illness and you are not actually sick.

While not everyone will experience this "flu," those who do report that it usually lasts several days to several weeks. The key is not to give up prematurely. This temporary feeling is simply your body transitioning from a carbohydrates-laden diet to a fat-laden diet. Keep in mind that you are altering your cell's metabolic processes for the better, so be patient with your body. It is trying to correct itself, so give it a break while it does its thing.

You will get over these symptoms (if you even experience them) and then you will feel energetic once again. To prepare yourself as much as possible to prevent yourself from getting the keto flu, here's what you can do:

♦ Transition into the keto diet slowly (i.e., eliminate carbohydrates slowly or add a few back if you took them all out).

♦ Increase your salt intake, which you can easily do with bone broth or by simply adding sea salt to your foods.

♦ Eat more fat. Adding MCT oil (or another fat) to your diet can help increase your blood ketones, which will help you feel more satiated and increase your mental clarity.

♦ Stay well hydrated because during this period of keto adaptation, we tend to lose more electrolytes.

♦ Take it easy. Do your best to relax and reduce stress.

♦ While you should not engage in vigorous physical activity, a good walk or hike can do wonders for your mental health.

make it easier? Meal planning is especially useful if you have children or an intense job, work night shifts, or are just plain busy.

Shopping for all your ingredients on Saturday and prepping them all on Sunday is a common practice, but everyone's life is different and there is no set schedule. Having lots of keto-approved foods in your pantry and freezer and buying fresh foods every few days is probably the easiest and most economical keto strategy. The first shopping list is included on page 30.

Easy Meals

Some of my favorite meals take only 10 to 15 minutes and are truly delicious. One of my most beloved meals is roast salmon, which pairs extremely well with raw or lightly steamed spinach. It's filling, it's delicious, and it's easy to make in about 20 minutes with few to no utensils necessary. Any fatty fish will keep well in the refrigerator, making it ideal for meal-planning purposes. Chicken is another protein that will not spoil quickly and is great for meal preparation. Some people think chicken is boring, so the key is mastering a few different types of marinades.

The beauty of the keto diet is that it frees your mind of clutter. Just remember to choose a protein, a little carbohydrate in the form of vegetables, and a good amount of fat.

Cook in Bulk

Have you ever seen economy-size packages of turkey, chicken, beef, pork, eggs, and fish? You may have thought you would never need so much food all at once, but guess what? Meal planning and prepping requires you to buy in bulk so you can cook in bulk—that way you have a meal ready when it's time to eat! Healthy oils, such as avocado, olive, and MCT, are also available in large containers, and you can find bulk produce like spinach, asparagus, green beans, broccoli, cauliflower, artichokes, tomatoes, and avocados at some stores.

Use Your Leftovers

You know that pork chop you didn't finish yesterday? Don't let it go to waste. Chop up the leftovers and throw them in a skillet with some cooking fat, garlic, onions, and sliced bell peppers. Add a splash of tamari sauce to the mix along with a sprinkle of sesame seeds and you have a whole new meal created out of something you didn't finish eating the day before.

You'll notice that I didn't tell you to just eat what you didn't finish the day before with no additions. That can easily lead to food boredom. Creating something new from your leftovers is the key to success. Remember, the keto diet does not have to be repetitive or boring; on the contrary, it can allow you to be extremely resourceful and imaginative.

When you prepare your meals in advance, it's always a good idea to cook a little more than you might need, in case you find yourself in a bind.

Setting Up Your Kitchen

There is a saying that "happiness is a well-stocked kitchen" and, honestly, there is a lot of truth to this. If you don't have anything in your house to eat, or nothing looks good to eat, you will most likely forget everything you have read thus far and settle for an unhealthy quick fix. Make sure that doesn't happen by always keeping your kitchen fully stocked with yummy keto items.

Refrigerated Items
These are great to have on hand for snacks.

- Eggs
- Fish or seafood (salmon, scallops, shrimp, cod, clams, etc.)
- Plain or unsweetened Greek yogurt or cottage cheese
- Sugar-free/nitrate-free, and free-range pork or beef sausages
- Sugar-free/nitrate-free turkey, pork, beef, and/or salmon bacon
- Sugar-free/nitrate-free chicken, turkey, ham, or beef deli meats

A note on meat and dairy: Always strive to use grass-fed and -finished meats as well as dairy products and eggs that come from animals that have had a grass-fed diet instead of a grain diet. For all meat and animal products, strive to buy free-range, as well.

Other Perishable Items

These will be good additions to a snack or a meal.

Asparagus	Green Beans	Pasture-raised, full-fat dairy and animal fats, such as tallow	Spinach
Avocados	Jicama		Tomatoes
Bell Peppers	Lemons/limes		
Eggplant	Mushrooms		

Pantry Items

These are essentials either on their own or to enhance whatever you pair them with.

- Canned chicken (without sugar)
- Canned coconut milk, tomatoes, olives, and artichokes
- Canned seafood/fish (tuna, sardines, salmon, clams, oysters, trout, etc.)
- Cocoa powder
- Jicama chips (like Jica Chips)
- Nori sheets (like SeaSnax, made with olive oil)
- Nut and seed flours
- Oils/fats: plant oils such as olive, avocado, almond, and macadamia nut, MCT oil, and animal fats such as ghee
- Sugar-free meat sticks/jerky
- Swerve sweetener, erythritol-sweetened syrups, stevia

A Word on Sweeteners

I like varying the keto-friendly sweeteners I use, so you should feel free to do so, as well. That said, the macros in this book are calculated using erythritol for consistency and ease. Erythritol is a sugar alcohol that does not spike blood sugar and has a glycemic index of zero. It is absorbed by the small intestine, but 90 percent is never metabolized, so it does not affect blood sugar. So while 1 teaspoon of erythritol has 4 grams of carbs, when calculating, you subtract 4 grams of the sugar alcohols, leaving you with zero net carbs.

Special Ingredients and Keto Brands

Your pantry and refrigerator are about to look remarkably different from how they once did thanks to the many special ingredients on the market to enhance the keto diet. Some of these may make you tilt your head and question my sanity, but please don't knock 'em before you try 'em! In fact, I do hope you embrace them, because a lot of these "weirdos" are used in the recipes within this book!

- Almond flour wraps
- Aquafaba
- Avocado oil
- Barlean's Butter Flavored Coconut Oil
- Bone broth
- Chia seeds
- ChocZero sugar-free syrups
- Chomps Meat Sticks, Nick's Sticks, Paleovalley Beef Sticks, and Sophia's Survival Food
- Coconut aminos
- Coconut oil and coconut butter
- Coconut wraps
- Collagen
- Designer Protein Totally Egg Protein Powders, Dutch Chocolate and Classic Vanilla
- Erythritol, stevia, and monk fruit extract
- Flax milk
- Flax oil
- Flaxseeds and flax meal
- G Hughes Sugar-Free BBQ Sauce
- Ghee
- Glucomannan
- Grass-fed/-finished whey protein
- Hemp milk
- Heinz No Sugar Added Ketchup
- Jica Chips, jicama chips
- Keto Queen Kreations baking mixes
- Jicama wraps
- Lakanto monk-fruit-extract sweetened syrups and chocolate
- Lily's sugar-free dark chocolate chips
- MCT oil
- Miracle Noodle shirataki noodles
- Mt. Olive No Sugar Added Bread & Butter Chips
- Natural Heaven hearts of palm pasta
- Nature's Hollow xylitol-sweetened syrups and honey
- NuCo Coconut Wraps
- NuNaturals stevia and stevia-sweetened syrups
- Nutritional yeast
- One on One flavor extracts

- Prymal Coffee Creamer
- Primal Kitchen avocado oil mayonnaise
- Primal Kitchen Collagen Fuel protein powders
- Psyllium husk
- SeaSnax seaweed chips
- So Delicious no-sugar-added coconut milk ice creams
- So Delicious unsweetened coconut milk
- SweetLeaf Liquid Stevia
- Swerve Granular, Swerve Confectioners, and Brown Swerve sweeteners (erythritol)
- Tahini
- Tallow
- Tamari sauce
- Teton Waters Ranch and Applegate grass-fed/-finished all-beef hot dogs
- The Good Chocolate Suger-Free Chocolate
- The Real Coconut coconut chips
- The Sprinkles Company Sugar-Free Sprinkles
- Unsweetened cocoa powder
- Xanthan gum

The 21-Day Meal Plan

Let's eat! You might be feeling a little clueless about where to start, but that's why I created this three-week meal plan. One of the biggest challenges when starting keto is figuring out how to add more fat to your diet. The meal plan in this chapter and the recipes that follow will help you meet your daily goal.

Notes Before You Begin

- These meal plans are for people who are looking to maintain their current weight. You can still follow these meal plans to lose weight—you'll simply need to cut your portion sizes. Combining these with intermittent fasting could do more in that regard, and you'll see I've already suggested which meals you can skip if you'd like.

- All of the meals listed use recipes from this book, so don't be overwhelmed if you have no idea what Meat Waffles/Bagels (page 52) are at first glance!

- Feel free to substitute any protein if you are not a fan of what's in the recipe, but remember that not all protein is created equal. So if a recipe calls for 6 ounces of salmon, feel free to use tuna; but keep in mind that their fat compositions are different, and you may need to add more fat to the tuna to meet your goal.

The Deal with Snacks

Personally, I don't find the need to snack very much thanks to the high fat content of my diet. These meals will successfully satisfy you. However, once in a while, you may need a snack. Just pay attention to the type of snack you're consuming, because it could mess with your macronutrient ratios. Alternatively, snacks can help you get in better macro balance. For instance, if you cook a particular meal with nonstick cooking spray instead of butter, ghee, macadamia nut oil, etc., you're going to be low in fat that day. Consuming almonds, full-fat cheese, or a little sugar-free dark chocolate as a snack will get you back into the right fat percentage.

Week One

MONDAY

MEAL 1: Coconut Flour–Based Chocolate Chip Waffles (page 51)

MEAL 2: Mayo-Less Tuna Salad (page 124)

MEAL 3: Meatloaf Muffins (page 137) (double recipe)

Macronutrients: Fat: 70%; Protein: 15%; Carbs: 15%

TUESDAY

MEAL 1: Eggs Benedict on Grilled Portobello Mushroom Caps (page 54) (if practicing intermittent fasting, skip this meal)

> **Easier Option:** 2 eggs scrambled with 3 slices of sugar-free ham (diced) and ½ green bell pepper (diced)

MEAL 2: Roasted Vegetable Salad (page 87)

MEAL 3: Chorizo Sliders (cook in bulk) (page 160) with beef bacon and Guacamole (page 210)

Macronutrients: Fat 70%; Protein 17%; Carbs 13%

WEDNESDAY

MEAL 1: Meatloaf Muffins (page 137) (leftovers)

MEAL 2: Turkey-Stuffed Avocados (page 143)

MEAL 3: Roasted Brussels Sprouts & Poached Eggs (page 108)

Macronutrients: Fat: 70%; Protein: 20%; Carbs: 10%

THURSDAY

MEAL 1: Breakfast Bowl with Cauliflower Hash (page 59) (include Breakfast Sausage, page 58)

MEAL 2: Minestrone Soup (page 90) (cook in bulk) with Cauliflower Popcorn (page 67)

> **Easier Option:** Bone Broth (page 203) mixed with precooked chicken and raw or steamed cauliflower

MEAL 3: Grilled Steak with Chimichurri (page 157) (cook in bulk; if practicing intermittent fasting, skip this meal)

Macronutrients: Fat 74%; Protein 16%; Carbs 10%

FRIDAY

MEAL 1: Scotch Eggs (page 71)

MEAL 2: Niçoise Salad (page 80)

MEAL 3: Fettuccine Alfredo (page 111) (double recipe)

Macronutrients: Fat: 75%; Protein: 18%; Carbs: 7%

SATURDAY

MEAL 1: Avocado "Toast" (page 141)

MEAL 2: Fettuccine Alfredo (page 111) (leftovers)

MEAL 3: Beef Burgers with Bacon (page 172)

Macronutrients: Fat 75%; Protein 18%; Carbs 7%

SUNDAY

MEAL 1: Sweet Egg Salad (page 186) or Coffee Cake (page 61) (if practicing intermittent fasting, skip this meal)

MEAL 2: Beef Stroganoff (page 175) (cook in bulk)

> **Easier Option:** 6 to 8 ounces of ground beef sautéed with onion and hearts of palm noodles

MEAL 3: Salmon with Mustard Sauce (page 120)

Macronutrients: Fat 70%; Protein 17%; Carbs 13%

SNACKS

Avocados, nuts, olives, sugar-free meat sticks, full-fat cheese sticks, canned fish, seaweed snacks, nitrate-free deli meat

Week 1 Shopping List

CANNED AND BOTTLED ITEMS

- Barbecue sauce, sugar-free
- Butternut squash or pumpkin, puréed, 1 (15-ounce) can
- Capers, 1 (8-ounce) jar
- ChocoZero syrup
- Coconut cream, heavy, 1 (13.5-ounce) can
- Coconut milk, full-fat, 1 (13.5-ounce) can
- Coconut milk, unsweetened, 1 (13.5-ounce) can
- Coconut oil, butter-flavored, 1 (32-ounce) jar

- Ginger, sugar-free pickled, 1 (12-ounce) jar
- Hearts of palm linguine, 2 (14-ounce) cans
- Hot sauce, sugar-free
- Ketchup, sugar-free
- Mayonnaise
- Mayonnaise, chipotle-lime, 1 (8-ounce) jar (optional)
- MCT oil, 1 (32-ounce) jar (optional)
- Mustard
- Olives, 1 (4.5-ounce) can
- Olives, Niçoise, 1 jar
- Pickle relish, sugar-free, 1 jar

- Pickles, sugar-free, 1 jar
- Tahini, 1 jar
- Tamari or coconut aminos
- Tomatoes, 1 (15-ounce) can
- Tomatoes, minced, 1 jar
- Tomatoes, sun-dried, 1 (8-ounce) jar
- Tomato paste, 1 (6-ounce) can
- Tuna, packed in olive oil, 1 (5-ounce) can
- Wine, white, 1 bottle

DAIRY AND EGGS

- Butter (1 pound) or coconut butter, 1 (14-ounce) jar
- Cheese, Parmesan, 8 ounces
- Cheese, pepper Jack, 8 ounces

- Cheese, soft, goat, 8 ounces
- Eggs, 1 to 2 dozen
- Ghee, 1 jar
- Heavy (whipping) cream, 1 pint
- Milk: coconut, almond, or full-fat dairy, 1 container

- So Delicious no-sugar-added coconut milk ice cream, 1 pint
- Yogurt, Greek, sugar-free, plain
- Yogurt, unsweetened, coconut

FROZEN FOODS

- Butternut squash, cubed, 1 to 2 (12-ounce) bags
- Cauliflower rice, 2 to 3 (12-ounce) bags
- Onions and peppers, 1 bag

MEAT

- Anchovy fillets, 6 (optional)
- Bacon, beef or pork, sugar-free, 1 package
- Beef bones, 3 to 5 pounds
- Beef, ground, 3 pounds (buy in bulk and freeze)
- Beef steak, 1 pound (buy in bulk and freeze)
- Beef tenderloin, 2 pounds (buy in bulk and freeze)
- Black cod, 1 pound (optional)
- Chicken, breasts and thighs, 1½ to 2 pounds (buy in bulk and freeze)
- Chicken tenders, 1 pound
- Game, 2 (6-ounce) steaks, beef, lamb, elk, venison, or bison
- Pork, ground, 1 pound (buy in bulk and freeze)
- Pork, tenderloin, 1½ pounds
- Salmon, tuna, or albacore, sushi-grade, ½ pound
- Sea bass (or any other fish), 2 whole, 2 pounds
- Turkey, ground, 1 pound
- Turkey, roasted, 8 ounces
- Turkey sausage

PANTRY ITEMS

- Allspice
- Almond flour
- Almond meal
- Apple cider vinegar
- Arrowroot flour
- Balsamic vinegar
- Basil, dried
- Bay leaves, dried
- Beef broth, 1 (32-ounce) container
- Black pepper
- Cayenne pepper
- Chicken broth, 1 container
- Chili powder
- Cinnamon
- Coriander
- Cumin
- Dill, dried
- Erythritol
- Fennel seeds
- Garlic powder
- Ginger, ground
- Marjoram, dried
- Mustard, Dijon
- Mustard powder
- Nonstick cooking spray
- Nutmeg
- Oil: avocado, coconut, olive, and sesame
- Onion powder
- Oregano, dried
- Paprika, dried
- Parsley, dried
- Red pepper flakes
- Rosemary, dried
- Sage, dried
- Salt
- Sesame seeds
- Sumac, ground
- Thyme, dried
- Turmeric
- Vanilla extract
- Vegetable broth, 1 container
- White pepper
- White wine vinegar

PRODUCE

- Asparagus, 1 bunch
- Avocados, 5
- Bell peppers,
  2 green, 4 red
- Brussels sprouts,
  1 (1 to 2 pounds) bag
- Cabbage, 2 heads
- Carrots, 2
- Cauliflower, 3 heads
- Celery, 1 to 2 bunches
- Chives, 1 bunch
- Cilantro, 2 bunches
- Cucumbers, 3
- Eggplant, 1
- Fennel, 1 bulb
- Garlic, 2 bulbs
- Green beans,
  1 (10-ounce) bag

- Jalapeño pepper,
  1 small
- Jicama, 1 bulb
- Kale
- Kohlrabi, 1 head
- Leek, 1
- Lemons, 5
- Lettuce, butter,
  1 (8-ounce) bag
- Lettuce mix, 2
  (10-ounce) bags
- Lime, 1
- Mushrooms, button
- Mushrooms, portobello,
  2 large, 8 small
- Onions, red and
  white, 10
- Oregano, 1 bunch

- Parsley, 3 bunches
- Pumpkin, fresh,
  1 medium
- Pumpkin, puréed,
  1 (15-ounce) can (NOT
  pumpkin pie mix)
- Salad greens,
  1 (10-ounce) bag
- Spaghetti squash, 1 or 2
- Spinach, 1
  (1-pound) bag
- Summer squash, 1
- Tomatoes, 3 to 5
- Tomatoes, cherry,
  ½ pint
- Tomatoes, plum, 2
- Zucchini, 1

OTHER

- Baking stevia, 1 bag
- Bread,
  keto-approved, 1 loaf
- Chocolate chips,
  sugar-free dark, 1 bag
- Coconut flour, 1 bag
- Coconut or almond flour
  wraps (1 to 3 packages)
- Coffee, decaf or regular

- Collagen, 1 container
- Flax meal, 1 bag
- Gelatin, 1 package
- Lemon juice, 1 container
- Lime juice, 1 container
- Miracle Noodle
  ziti-shaped noodles,
  1 (7-ounce) bag
- Nori sheets, 1 package

- Nutritional yeast, 1 bag
- Protein powder,
  coconut-vanilla or
  vanilla, 1 container
- Seaweed mix, 1 bag
- Shirataki noodles,
  2 packages
- Wasabi (optional)

These shopping lists may look rather intimidating, but don't be alarmed. You likely already have some of these ingredients in your pantry, and if not, you will have leftover ingredients you can use in the coming weeks. Also, a lot of these meats you can buy in bulk and freeze. Just don't forget to plan in advance and thaw them accordingly.

Week Two

MONDAY

MEAL 1: Deviled Eggs (page 64) with grilled asparagus (if practicing intermittent fasting, skip this meal)

MEAL 2: Niçoise Salad (page 80)

MEAL 3: Beef Stroganoff (page 175)

Easier Option: Grilled or pan-seared salmon drizzled with olive oil and paired with spaghetti squash (Trader Joe's has precut spaghetti squash that just needs to be microwaved)

Macronutrients: Fat 70%; Protein 25%; Carbs 5%

TUESDAY

MEAL 1: Avocado "Toast" (page 141)

MEAL 2: Mayo-Less Tuna Salad (page 124)

MEAL 3: Chicken Shawarma (page 133) (double recipe)

Macronutrients: Fat 72%; Protein 23%; Carbs 5%

WEDNESDAY

MEAL 1: Lemon–Poppy Seed Muffins (page 77)

MEAL 2: Chicken Shawarma (page 133) (leftovers)

MEAL 3: Pork Tacos/Burrito Wraps (page 158) with Guacamole (page 210) (double the Guacamole recipe)

Macronutrients: Fat: 70%; Protein: 18%; Carbs: 12%

THURSDAY

MEAL 1: Eggs Benedict on Grilled Portobello Mushroom Caps (page 54)

MEAL 2: Pork Tacos/Burrito Wraps (page 158) with Guacamole (page 210) (leftovers) (if practicing intermittent fasting, skip this meal)

MEAL 3: Fettuccine Alfredo (page 111) (double recipe)

Macronutrients: Fat: 71%; Protein: 16%; Carbs: 13%

FRIDAY

MEAL 1: Coconut Flour–Based Chocolate Chip Waffles (page 51)

MEAL 2: Fettuccine Alfredo (page 111) (leftovers)

MEAL 3: Meatloaf Muffins (page 137) (double recipe)

Macronutrients: Fat 71%; Protein 13%; Carbs 16%

SATURDAY

MEAL 1: Breakfast Bowl with Cauliflower Hash (page 59)

MEAL 2: Meatloaf Muffins (page 137) (leftovers)

MEAL 3: Cobb Salad (page 92)

Macronutrients: Fat 70%; Protein 22%; Carbs 8%

SUNDAY

MEAL 1: Scotch Eggs (page 71)

MEAL 2: Turkey-Stuffed Avocados (page 143)

MEAL 3: Beef Burgers with Bacon (page 172) (double recipe)

Macronutrients: Fat 72%; Protein 22%; Carbs 6%

SNACKS

Nuts and seeds, kale chips, hard-boiled eggs, bacon, pork rinds, Epic Bars, veggie sticks and Guacamole (page 210)

Week 2 Shopping List

CANNED AND BOTTLED ITEMS

- Artichoke hearts, 1 to 2 cans
- Capers, 1 (8-ounce) jar
- ChocoZero syrup
- Ginger, sugar-free pickled, 1 (6-ounce) jar
- Hot sauce, sugar-free

- Ketchup, sugar-free
- Mayonnaise
- Mustard
- Olives, black or Niçoise, 1 can
- Salmon or tuna, packed in olive oil, 1 or 2 (5-ounce) cans

- Salmon or tuna, packed in water, 1 (5-ounce) can
- Tamari or coconut aminos
- Tomatoes, sun-dried, 1 (8-ounce) jar
- Tuna, packed in olive oil, 1 (5-ounce) can

DAIRY AND EGGS

- Butter
- Cheese of choice
- Eggs, 1 to 2 dozen

- Ghee, 1 jar
- So Delicious no-sugar-added coconut milk ice cream, 1 pint

- Yogurt, Greek, sugar-free, plain
- Yogurt, unsweetened, coconut

FROZEN FOODS

- Cauliflower rice, 2 to 3 (12-ounce) bags

- Green beans, 1 (12-ounce) bag

- Onions and peppers, 1 (12-ounce) bag

MEAT

- Anchovy fillets, 6 (optional)
- Bacon, sugar-free, 1 package
- Beef tenderloin, 2 pounds
- Beef, ground, 1 pound
- Beef steak, 1 pound
- Chicken, breast or thigh

- Pork chops, 1 to 2 pounds (buy in bulk and freeze)
- Pork, ground, 1 to 2 pounds
- Pork, tenderloin, 1½ pounds
- Salmon belly, skin-on, 1 pound

- Sausage, sugar-free chicken, 1 package
- Tuna, ahi, 1 (8- to 12-ounce) steak
- Turkey, ground, 1 to 2 pounds
- Turkey, roasted, 8 ounces

PANTRY ITEMS

- Allspice
- Almond flour
- Arrowroot flour
- Basil, dried

- Beef broth, 1 to 2 (32-ounce) containers
- Black pepper
- Cinnamon
- Coconut flour, 1 bag

- Coffee, decaf or regular
- Erythritol
- Fennel seeds
- Garlic powder
- Marjoram, dried

- MCT oil, 1 (32-ounce) jar (optional)
- Mustard, Dijon
- Mustard, spicy
- Nutmeg
- Oil: algae, avocado, coconut, olive, and sesame
- Onion powder
- Oregano, dried
- Paprika, dried
- Red pepper flakes
- Red wine vinegar
- Sage, dried
- Salt
- Sumac, ground
- Thyme, dried
- Vanilla extract
- Vegetable broth, 1 (32-ounce) container
- White pepper
- White wine vinegar

PRODUCE

- Asparagus, 3 to 4 bunches
- Avocados, 3
- Brussels sprouts, 1 pound
- Cabbage, 1 head
- Carrots, 1 bunch
- Cauliflower, 2 heads
- Celery, 1 bunch
- Cilantro, 2 bunches
- Cucumbers, 1 to 2
- Eggplant, 3
- Fennel, 1 bulb
- Garlic, 1 bulb
- Gingerroot, 1
- Jicama, 1 bulb
- Kohlrabi, 1 head
- Leeks, 1 or 2
- Lettuce, butter, 2 heads
- Lettuce, iceberg, 1 head
- Lettuce, romaine, 1 to 2 heads
- Mushrooms, button, one pack
- Mushrooms, cremini, one pack
- Mushrooms, portobello, 2 large, 8 small
- Onions, 3 to 4
- Parsley, 1 bunch
- Pumpkin, puréed, 1 (15-ounce) can (NOT pumpkin pie mix)
- Salad greens, mixed
- Scallions, 2 to 3 bunches
- Spinach, 1 (1-pound) bag
- Tomatoes, 2 to 4
- Tomatoes, cherry, 1 to 2 pints
- Zucchini, 2

OTHER

- Baking powder
- Baking stevia, 1 bag
- Chia seeds (optional)
- Chocolate chips, sugar-free dark
- Collagen
- Coconut wraps, 1 package
- Lemon juice, 1 container
- Lime juice, 1 container
- Nutritional yeast
- Poppy seeds
- Shirataki noodles, 1 to 3 (7-ounce) packages (buy in bulk)
- Protein powder, keto-approved, 1 container

Week Three

MONDAY

MEAL 1: Cauliflower 'N' Oatmeal (page 50)

MEAL 2: Beef Burgers with Bacon (page 172) (leftovers) with Avocado Fries (page 75)

MEAL 3: Chopped Bitter Greens Salad (page 89) with cooked chicken breast and Dairy-Free White Chocolate Bark (page 180)

Macronutrients: Fat 75%; Protein 15%; Carbs 10%

TUESDAY

MEAL 1: Roasted Brussels Sprouts & Poached Eggs (page 108)

MEAL 2: Meatloaf Muffins (page 137) with Eggplant Chips (page 72)

MEAL 3: Chicken Teriyaki (page 131) with cauliflower rice (if practicing intermittent fasting, skip this meal)

Macronutrients: Fat 70%; Protein 21%; Carbs 9%

WEDNESDAY

MEAL 1: Lemon–Poppy Seed Muffins (page 77)

MEAL 2: Meatloaf Muffins (page 137) with Cauliflower Popcorn (page 67) (if practicing intermittent fasting, skip this meal)

MEAL 3: Almond Meal–Crusted Chicken Fingers (page 135) (double recipe) with Avocado Fries (page 75)

Macronutrients: Fat 70%; Protein 20%; Carbs 10%

THURSDAY

MEAL 1: Breakfast Bowl with Cauliflower Hash (page 59)

MEAL 2: Mayo-Less Tuna Salad (page 124) with Hot Cocoa/Chocolate Milk (page 205)

MEAL 3: Almond Meal–Crusted Chicken Fingers (page 135) (leftovers) with Asian Cucumber Salad (page 94)

Macronutrients: Fat 70%; Protein 20%; Carbs 10%

FRIDAY

MEAL 1: Avocado "Toast" (page 141) (if practicing intermittent fasting, skip this meal)

MEAL 2: Halibut Curry (page 129) (warmed in hollowed-out bell peppers)

MEAL 3: Fettuccine Alfredo (page 111) (double recipe) with broccoli

Macronutrients: Fat 71%; Protein 20%; Carbs 9%

SATURDAY

MEAL 1: Eggs Benedict on Grilled Portobello Mushroom Caps (page 54)

MEAL 2: Niçoise Salad (page 80)

MEAL 3: Fettuccine Alfredo (page 111) (leftovers)

Macronutrients: Fat 61%; Protein 32%; Carbs 7%

SUNDAY

MEAL 1: Coconut Flour–Based Chocolate Chip Waffles (page 51)

MEAL 2: Turkey-Stuffed Avocados (page 143)

MEAL 3: Pork Tacos/Burrito Wraps (page 158) with Dairy-Free White Chocolate Bark (page 180)

Macronutrients: Fat 70%; Protein 14%; Carbs 16%

SNACKS

Sugar-free dark chocolate, sugar-free flavored coconut butter, leftover vegetables drizzled with MCT oil, sugar- and nitrate-free hot dogs, sugar-free smoked salmon, pickles, nut butter, jicama chips (like Jica Chips)

Week 3 Shopping List

CANNED AND BOTTLED ITEMS

- Anchovies, packed in olive oil, 1 (2-ounce) can
- Artichoke hearts, 2 cans
- Barbecue sauce, sugar-free
- Capers, 1 (8-ounce) jar
- ChocoZero syrup
- Cinnamon maple syrup, sugar-free

- Coconut milk, full-fat, 1 (13.5-ounce) can
- Ginger, sugar-free pickled, 1 (6-ounce) jar
- Hot sauce, sugar-free
- Ketchup, sugar-free
- Mustard
- Olives, 1 (4.5-ounce) can
- Olives, Niçoise, 1 jar
- Sardines, 1 can

- Stock, seafood, 1 (32-ounce) container
- Tamari or coconut aminos
- Tomatoes, sun-dried, 1 (8-ounce) jar
- Tomato sauce, keto-approved, 1 jar
- Tuna, packed in olive oil, 1 (5-ounce) can

DAIRY AND EGGS

- Almond or coconut milk, unsweetened, 1 container
- Butter or ghee, 1 pound
- Cheese: Cheddar, Parmesan, and Romano

- Coconut milk, unsweetened, 1 container
- Eggs, 1 to 2 dozen
- Heavy (whipping) cream, 1 pint
- Milk, flax, unsweetened

- Milk, full-fat
- So Delicious no-sugar-added coconut milk ice cream, 1 pint
- Yogurt, unsweetened, coconut

FROZEN FOOD

- Butternut squash, cubed, 1 to 2 (12-ounce) bags

- Cauliflower rice, 2 to 3 bags

MEAT

- Anchovy fillets, 6 (optional)
- Bacon, sugar-free, 1 package
- Beef brisket, 1 to 3 pounds
- Beef, ground
- Chicken breasts and thighs (buy in bulk and freeze)

- Chicken tenders, 2 pounds
- Halibut or other whitefish, 1 to 2 pounds
- Pork, ground, 1 pound
- Pork, tenderloin, 1½ pounds

- Salmon, sushi-grade, 1 to 2 pounds
- Tuna, ahi, 1 pound
- Turkey, ground, 1 to 2 pounds
- Turkey, roasted, 8 ounces
- Turkey, sliced deli meat, 8 ounces

PANTRY ITEMS

- Allspice
- Almond or coconut flour (optional)
- Almond meal, 1 package
- Apple cider vinegar
- Black pepper
- Basil, dried
- Cayenne pepper
- Cilantro, dried
- Cinnamon, ground
- Cookie/cake flavor extract (optional)
- Cumin, ground
- Curry powder
- Erythritol
- "Everything bagel" spice
- Flax meal
- Garlic powder
- Ginger, ground
- Kebab seasoning
- Marjoram, dried
- MCT oil, 1 (32-ounce) jar (optional)
- Mustard, Dijon
- Nonstick cooking spray
- Nordic Naturals Omega-3 oil, lemon flavored
- Nutmeg
- Oil: algae, avocado, coconut, olive, macadamia nut, or sesame
- Onion powder
- Oregano, dried
- Paprika, dried
- Red pepper flakes
- Rosemary, dried
- Saffron, ground
- Sage, dried
- Salt
- Sesame seeds
- Sumac, ground
- Thyme, dried
- Turmeric, ground
- Vanilla extract
- White pepper
- White wine vinegar
- Xanthan gum, 1 package

PRODUCE

- Arugula, 1 bag
- Asparagus, 2 to 3 bunches
- Avocados, 3 to 5
- Basil, 2 bunches
- Bell peppers, 1 green, 1 red
- Broccoli, 1 head
- Brussels sprouts, 1 pound
- Butternut squash, 1
- Cabbages, 1 green head, 1 red head
- Carrots, 1 bunch
- Cauliflower, 1 head
- Celery, 1 bunch
- Celery root, 1
- Chives, 1 bunch
- Cilantro, 2 bunches
- Cucumbers, 2 large
- Dandelion greens, 1 bunch
- Eggplant, 2
- Endive, 1 head
- Fennel, 1 or 2 bulbs
- Garlic, 1 bulb
- Green beans, 1 (10-ounce) bag
- Jalapeño pepper, 1
- Jicama, 1 bulb
- Kale
- Kohlrabi, 1 head
- Leek, 1 bunch
- Lettuce, butter, 1 (8-ounce) bag
- Mushrooms, 1 container
- Mushrooms, button 1 container
- Mushrooms, portobello, 2 large, 8 small
- Onions, 5
- Parsley, 1 bunch
- Parsley, Italian, 1 bunch
- Radicchio, 1 head
- Shallots, 1 to 2

- Spaghetti squash, 1
- Spinach, 1 to 2 pounds

OTHER
- Baking powder
- Baking stevia, 1 bag
- Chocolate chips, sugar-free dark
- Chocolate, sugar-free dark, 1 (3-ounce) bar
- Cocoa powder, unsweetened, 1 package
- Coconut flour wraps, 1 package
- Lemon juice, 1 container
- Nori sheets, 1 package

- Tomatoes, 2 to 4
- Tomatoes, cherry, 1 (10-ounce) container

- Nutritional yeast
- Poppy seeds
- Protein powder, keto-approved, plain or vanilla, 1 container
- Psyllium husk powder
- Seaweed mix, 1 bag
- Shirataki noodles, 2 (7-ounce) packages
- Tofu, 1 (8-ounce) package

- Zucchini, 1

Tips for Building Your Own Plan

I have seen a lot of meal plans for the keto diet that suggest eating a tiny bit of chicken with a few tablespoons of butter and some steamed vegetables. To me, that sounds about as boring as waiting in a doctor's office for three hours without a cell phone. I want to excite you about keto so it's easy to make your own.

1. Determine your goals. Are you trying to lose or maintain weight? Once you know what you want, an online calculator can help you come up with a calorie goal that's appropriate for your body.

2. Hitting the right macro balance is the most important thing you can do for success. Again, find your ideal ratio using an online calculator. There are many different types, so I won't endorse one in particular here.

3. Use the snacks listed in the meal plan as you need them. Sometimes we miscalculate our food intake or we just feel a bit hungrier one day based on hormones or other factors. That's when these snacks come in handy—they're there to help you.

4. Don't be scared to eat out at restaurants. It's not as hard as you'd think—you just have be direct when ordering. For example, no bun, no French fries, an extra meat patty, or another slice of cheese. Be sure to ask what kind of fats they are using to cook your meal and what sauces the meats might have been marinated in. Be friendly but clear with your server about what you can't have.

5. Think outside the box. Again, boiled chicken, butter, and steamed vegetables sounds a little boring, I admit. But if you roast those vegetables, pan-sear that chicken in the butter, and add herbs and spices, you're going to excite your taste buds and make them to want to eat this way for the long haul.

At last, the entrée has arrived. It's time to dig into the recipe section of this book so you can get cooking.

Self-Kindness and Intuitive Eating

We typically get angry with ourselves when we eat something off-diet or eat more than planned, which can lead to a downward spiral where we feel totally defeated and say, "to hell with it." Here are a few tips that may come in handy if you veer off course.

♦ If you live with someone who is not on the keto lifestyle, tell them your goals and why you are eating keto so they can be supportive, and not undermine your pursuits.

♦ Create your own space in the kitchen where you can stock your food, so you never see the snacks and goodies in the house that are not keto-approved.

♦ Feeling stressed is a huge reason people eat off-diet. Before heading to the pantry, ask yourself if you are truly hungry or whether you are stressed. Then ask yourself what you're stressed about and why. Be honest with yourself. If you find that you're reaching for food because you're stressed, that's okay—don't feel bad about it. This is a habit most of us have. Take a few minutes to write a list of other ways you may be able to combat stress, such as calling a relative, getting a massage, going for a walk, or even just drinking some water.

♦ Let's say you ate keto all day but caved and ate French fries at dinner. Forgive yourself! Remember that it's all about transitioning, so slipping here and there is nothing to feel guilty over. Do your best to get back on track, and give yourself a pat on the back for committing to this new lifestyle in the first place. Even the most seasoned of us fall out of ketosis once in a while. You have the tools to get yourself right back into ketosis if you slip out of it.

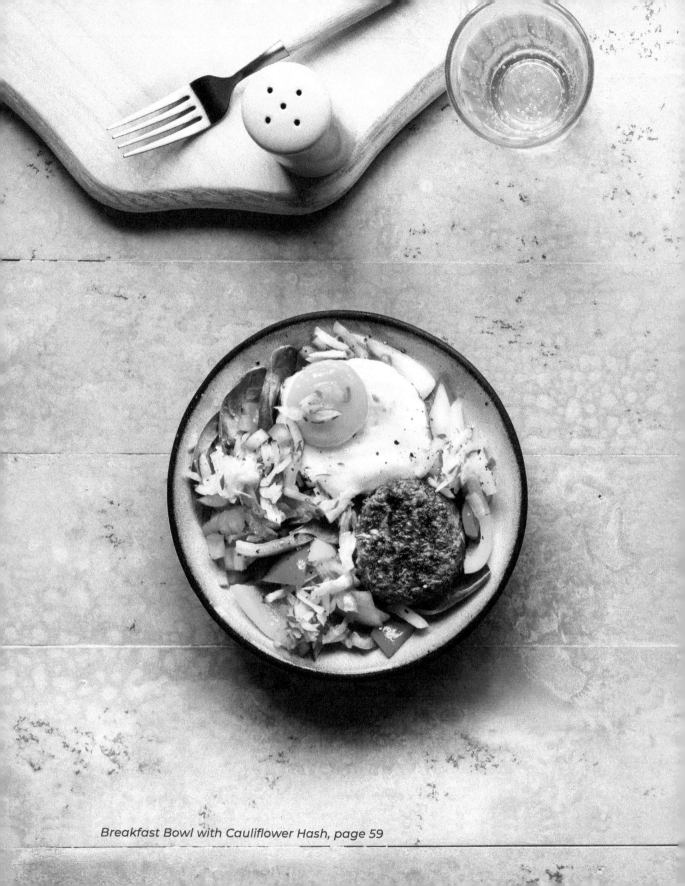

Breakfast Bowl with Cauliflower Hash, page 59

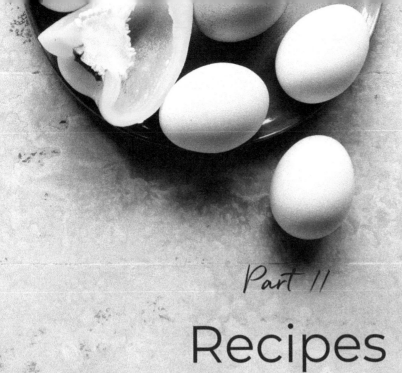

Part II

Recipes

We have finally arrived at the "meat" of this book. I put "meat" in quotes because in addition to meaty recipes you will find lots of scrumptious fish, poultry, egg, and vegetable recipes. What you won't find too much of are recipes comprised of dairy, soy, and nuts—and I promise you won't miss them! The best part is that these recipes will keep you satiated and satisfied for much longer than you are used to. This will enable you to get into ketosis without actually feeling like you are drastically reducing your calorie consumption.

You'll see that I've provided three kinds of labels for the recipes in order to help you out. They are:

Bulk Cook—you can cook large quantities and save some for later

One Pot—you only need one pot/pan/skillet for this recipe (not including mixing bowls, etc.)

Super Quick—takes 30 minutes or less, including prep time and cook time

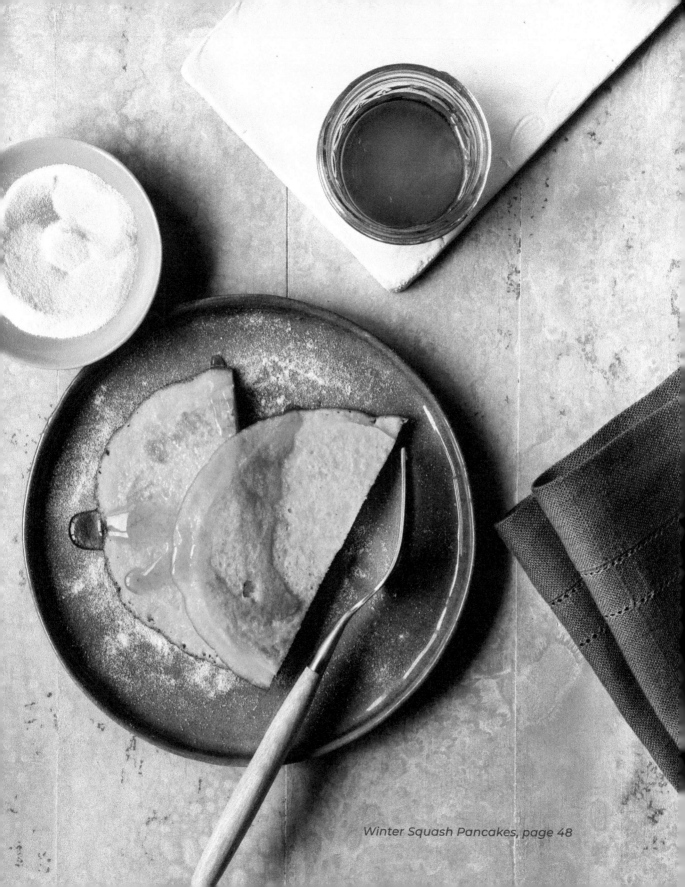

Winter Squash Pancakes, page 48

Chapter 3

Breakfast

Good morning! What'll you be having? Pancakes? Eggs Benedict? French toast, perhaps? And here you thought you couldn't eat foods like that on the keto diet. Grab a cup of black coffee spiked with some coconut oil or ghee, it's time to break that fast and chow down!

Winter Squash Pancakes 48

Brussels Sprouts & Ground Beef Scrambled Eggs 49

Cauliflower 'N' Oatmeal 50

Coconut Flour–Based Chocolate Chip Waffles 51

Meat Waffles/Bagels 52

Eggs Benedict on Grilled Portobello Mushroom Caps 54

French Toast 56

Breakfast Sausage 58

Breakfast Bowl with Cauliflower Hash 59

Coffee Cake 61

WINTER SQUASH PANCAKES

PREP TIME: 5 MINUTES / COOK TIME: 8 TO 10 MINUTES

I've set foot in a breakfast-style diner just once in my life, and it was to use the bathroom. I was desperate! Honestly, that's the only time I feel one should visit a restaurant like this because, really, you can make your own flapjacks at home with a quarter of the calories and zero trans-fatty acids (you know, those bad fats that wreak havoc on your cholesterol levels and negatively affect your heart health). This recipe for pancakes is full of potassium, magnesium, and boatloads of beta-carotene!

SUPER QUICK

1
SERVING

Per Serving: Calories: 331; Total Fat: 22g; Total Carbohydrates: 25g; Net Carbs: 17g; Fiber: 8g; Protein: 11g; Erythritol: 24g

Macronutrients: Fat 58%; Protein 13%; Carbs 28%

BRAND: *Swerve is a brand of erythritol sweetener that is very low in calories (lots of packages claim zero calories) and has no strange aftertaste. Erythritol also does not raise your blood sugar levels, which makes it a perfect sweetener for the keto diet.*

1 egg
½ cup puréed butternut squash
3 tablespoons coconut flour
2 tablespoons erythritol
¼ teaspoon vanilla extract
1 tablespoon coconut oil or butter
Powdered coffee creamer or maple syrup (optional)

1. In a mixing bowl, combine the egg, butternut squash, flour, erythritol, and vanilla and stir together.

2. In a small sauté pan over medium heat, melt the coconut oil or butter. Pour your batter in.

3. Cook one side of the pancake until you can easily stick your spatula underneath all sides, 5 to 8 minutes.

4. Carefully flip the pancake over and cook for another 3 to 4 minutes.

5. Remove from the pan and place your pancake on a plate. Drizzle powdered coffee creamer and/or maple syrup over the top, if desired.

TIP: *Coconut flour is very absorbent. It is best to leave it alone for a while to let it swell and absorb the egg and squash before cooking.*

BRUSSELS SPROUTS & GROUND BEEF SCRAMBLED EGGS

PREP TIME: 10 MINUTES / COOK TIME: 10 TO 15 MINUTES

It's interesting how most people hate Brussels sprouts when they're young but grow to love them. These tiny heads of cabbage are ridiculously healthy for you. They're rich in antioxidants and vitamin K, and they're delicious if cooked correctly. Eating Brussels sprouts roasted or stir-fried, as this recipe calls for, allows the true sweet flavor to shine. And if you're one of the people who still don't like them, this recipe may very well convert you!

1 tablespoon butter-flavored coconut oil

10 Brussels sprouts, halved

¼ pound ground beef (80 percent lean)

2 eggs, beaten

Salt

Freshly ground black pepper

Sugar-free hot sauce (optional)

1. In a sauté pan over medium-high heat, melt the coconut oil and then add the Brussels sprouts. Stir, then cover and cook for 3 to 5 minutes.

2. Add the ground beef and cook for another 3 to 5 minutes, stirring continuously.

3. Add the eggs, season with salt and pepper, and scramble everything together for 2 to 3 minutes.

4. Pour the mixture onto a plate and top with hot sauce, if you like things a bit spicier!

TIP: *If you don't want to go through the hassle of trimming and cleaning the Brussels sprouts, you may be able to find them frozen (read: already prepped) in the freezer section of your grocery store.*

SWAP: *You can use regular butter in this recipe. 1¼ tablespoons of butter has the same amount of fat grams as 1 tablespoon of coconut oil.*

SUPER QUICK

1
SERVING

Per Serving: Calories: 626; Total Fat: 46g; Total Carbohydrates: 18g; Net Carbs: 11g; Fiber: 7g; Protein: 38g

Macronutrients: Fat 66%; Protein 24%; Carbs 10%

BRAND: *Barlean's has the most delicious butter-flavored coconut oil—you will be convinced it's actually butter. Other brands that produce and sell butter-flavored coconut oils are Nutiva and Now Foods, which can all be found in stores or on amazon.com or iHerb.com.*

CAULIFLOWER 'N' OATMEAL

PREP TIME: 5 MINUTES / COOK TIME: 5 MINUTES

When I was a little kid, my mom used to let me eat instant oatmeal because she believed it to be the healthiest "evil" on the market; however, it has 12 grams of sugar in one tiny packet. And let's be real: I always had two or three packets of the sweet stuff. That's a whole lot of insulin-spiking sugar. With this recipe, though, you don't have to worry about that. This oatmeal-type recipe contains zero sugars and grains, yet retains all the sweetness you remember from that bowl of comfort food.

SUPER QUICK

1
SERVING

Per Serving: Calories: 242; Total Fat: 18g; Total Carbohydrates: 8g; Net Carbs: 5g; Fiber: 3g; Protein: 12g

Macronutrients: Fat 67%; Protein 20%; Carbs 13%

SWAP: *Use unsweetened almond milk or coconut milk in this recipe if you'd like; however, this will slightly change the macronutrients. You can instead use a protein powder (like grass-fed/-finished whey or egg protein), but, again, the macronutrients will differ from what's listed.*

1 cup frozen cauliflower (you can use raw, but the cooking time will be longer)

¼ cup unsweetened flax milk

1 scoop Primal Kitchen Collagen Fuel protein powder (Vanilla-Coconut or Chocolate)

½ tablespoon ground cinnamon

1 tablespoon coconut oil

Erythritol "brown sugar" or sugar-free syrup (optional)

1. In a blender, combine the cauliflower (if using raw, you will need to steam it first until fork-tender), flax milk, protein powder, cinnamon, and coconut oil and purée.

2. Transfer to a saucepan and warm over medium heat for about 5 minutes.

3. Remove from the heat, pour into a bowl, and sprinkle sweetener or sugar-free syrup on top, if desired.

TIP: *If you don't have a blender, not to worry! You can combine all of these ingredients in a bowl, mix together by hand, and then warm on the stove as the recipe instructions state. This will just lead to a chunkier "oatmeal" with a texture and mouthfeel you may end up liking more.*

COCONUT FLOUR–BASED CHOCOLATE CHIP WAFFLES

PREP TIME: 10 MINUTES / COOK TIME: 8 TO 10 MINUTES

If you're waffling back and forth trying to decide if you should buy premade waffles or make your own, remind yourself that those premade ones are nutritionally void while these coconut flour–based waffles are chock-full of healthy fat, antioxidants, and fiber.

½ cup coconut flour

3 tablespoons baking stevia

1 egg

½ cup unsweetened coconut yogurt

1 teaspoon vanilla extract

2 tablespoons sugar-free dark chocolate chips

1 tablespoon coconut oil, for greasing

1 scoop So Delicious no-sugar-added coconut milk ice cream

1 to 2 tablespoons ChocoZero, or syrup of choice

½ cup whipped cream or coconut whipped cream

1. Preheat a waffle iron.

2. In a bowl, mix together the flour, stevia, egg, yogurt, vanilla, and chocolate chips until well combined.

3. Grease the waffle iron well with coconut oil, butter, or nonstick spray. Pour in half the batter. Close and let cook for 8 to 10 minutes. (Check to make sure nothing is burning, and if it is, turn down the heat.)

4. Remove the waffle and transfer to a plate. Repeat step 3 with the remaining batter to make one more waffle, and transfer it to a separate plate when done cooking.

5. Scoop ½ cup of ice cream on top of each and drizzle the syrup over everything. Top each waffle with whipped cream.

TIP: *No waffle maker, no problem! Feel free to make pancakes instead. Using this batter, follow the instructions for the Winter Squash Pancakes (page 48).*

SUPER QUICK

2
SERVINGS

Per Serving: Calories: 582; Total Fat: 44g; Total Carbohydrates: 39g; Net Carbs: 20g; Fiber: 19g; Protein: 12g; Erythritol: 18g; Syrup Carbs: 15g

Macronutrients: Fat 68%; Protein 6%; Carbs 26%

SWAP: *You can use almond flour for this recipe, though you'll need 1 cup of almond flour for every ¼ cup coconut flour. (Coconut flour is far more absorbent than almond flour.)*

BRAND: *The sugar-free chocolate brands that I love are: Coco Polo, Lily's, Lakanto, The Good Chocolate, and Know Foods.*

MEAT WAFFLES/BAGELS

PREP TIME: 5 MINUTES / COOK TIME: 5 TO 20 MINUTES, DEPENDING
ON IF YOU MAKE WAFFLES OR BAGELS

If I ever wound up owning a food truck, mine would sell meat waffles and bagels. Perhaps I would call it Waffly Good Hole in One. Seriously, these are so good that after you try them, you're going to be contacting me, wondering how you can fund my business venture!

SUPER QUICK

4

SERVINGS

Per Serving: Calories: 294;
Total Fat: 19g; Total
Carbohydrates: 2g; Net Carbs:
2g; Fiber: 0g; Protein: 29g

Macronutrients: Fat 60%;
Protein 39%; Carbs 1%

Avocado oil, coconut oil, or butter, for greasing
1 pound ground beef, turkey, pork, or bison
½ tablespoon garlic powder
½ tablespoon dried oregano
½ tablespoon paprika
Salt
Freshly ground black pepper
4 eggs, sunny-side-up or over-easy, for serving (optional)
Sliced cheese, for serving (optional)
(You can use any other herbs/spices you like)

1. First, determine if you're making meat waffles or meat bagels. Once you figure that out, grab your waffle maker or your bagel baking dish. (If you have neither, perhaps you have a muffin tin? If you have one of those, then you can cook your meat the same way you would the bagels.) Grease the waffle maker or baking dish with oil or butter; if making bagels, preheat the oven to 380°F.

2. In a bowl, mix the meat with the garlic, oregano, paprika, salt, and pepper. Separate the meat mixture into 4 equal portions and press into the waffle maker or baking dish.

3. The meat will cook 3 to 5 minutes in your waffle maker or 15 to 20 minutes in the oven. (If you're cooking poultry, obviously you need to cook it until completely done.)

4. Once done cooking, let cool slightly, but they should still be slightly warm when you serve them.

5. When ready to serve, place a slice of cheese and an egg on top of each waffle, if desired, and poke the yolk for some extreme yolk porn. Slice the meat bagels in half and place a slice of cheese and an egg inside, if desired. Take a bite like you would a regular bagel, but, warning, yolk may dribble down your face!

TIP: *I highly recommend purchasing a bagel/doughnut pan and/or a waffle maker because it will help bring some variety to your keto diet.*

SWAP: *Get creative! Use any meat you'd like, or add bacon to your waffle or bagel for an extra flavor explosion.*

EGGS BENEDICT ON GRILLED PORTOBELLO MUSHROOM CAPS

PREP TIME: 5 MINUTES / COOK TIME: 10 TO 15 MINUTES

While it's not especially encouraged on the keto diet, every so often some of us need a drink! (Alcoholic recipes can be found in this book. See chapter 10.) And sometimes one drink leads to two, and two leads to three, which leads to a horrific hangover. What's a person to do? "Medicate" with hangover food, of course. Portobello mushrooms contain B vitamins, selenium, potassium, copper, and vitamin D (as do the eggs), so everything here will help you in feeling like yourself again!

SUPER QUICK

1

SERVING

Per Serving: Calories: 841;
Total Fat: 76g; Total
Carbohydrates: 14g;
Net Carbs: 9g; Fiber: 5g;
Protein: 32g

Macronutrients: Fat 80%;
Protein 14%; Carbs 6%

2 portobello mushroom caps
1 tablespoon avocado oil
2 large spinach leaves
2 slices bacon
2 eggs
1 egg yolk
¼ teaspoon freshly squeezed lemon juice
1½ tablespoons olive oil
Pinch salt
1 teaspoon paprika
Chopped fresh parsley, for serving
Sugar-free hot sauce, for serving (optional)

1. Preheat the oven to broil or to 400°F, or heat a grill.

2. Take a damp paper towel and wipe off the mushroom caps, removing any stem. Rub them all over with the avocado oil, place on a baking sheet, and broil or roast in the oven for 10 minutes, flipping them halfway through. Alternatively, you can grill the mushroom caps for about 5 minutes on each side.

3. In a skillet while the mushrooms are baking, fry the bacon (which doesn't need any added fat) to your desired doneness. Remove from skillet and set aside.

4. Remove the mushrooms from the oven or grill, transfer to a plate, and place the spinach leaves and bacon on top.

5. To poach the eggs, fill a saucepan with water and bring to a boil, then lower the heat to a simmer.

6. Crack the eggs into a small bowl and carefully pour them into the simmering water. Turn off the heat, cover the pan, and let the eggs cook for about 5 minutes.

7. Carefully remove the eggs from the pan with a slotted spoon, straining over the pan, and place on top of the crispy bacon, spinach, and mushroom caps.

8. In a blender, combine the egg yolk, lemon juice, olive oil, and salt. Turn on the blender to its lowest setting and let the mixture whip together.

9. When the hollandaise sauce looks creamy, turn off the blender and pour the sauce over your mushrooms topped with spinach, bacon, and eggs.

10. Sprinkle with the paprika, chopped parsley, and a dash or two of hot sauce, if desired.

SWAP: *Instead of portobello mushrooms, you can use grilled or roasted eggplant slices.*

FRENCH TOAST

PREP TIME: 10 TO 15 MINUTES / COOK TIME: 12 TO 30 MINUTES

I love French toast so much that I wish it was invented by my ancestors, so I could truly claim it. Did you know that French toast isn't even really French? The traditional recipe actually dates back to the Roman Empire. That said, this specific recipe is, in fact, French because I am French, and I invented it. So dreams can come true.

3
SERVINGS

Per Serving: Calories: 506;
Total Fat: 34g;
Total Carbohydrates: 26g; Net
Carbs: 17g; Fiber: 9g; Protein:
24g; Erythritol Carbs: 21g

Macronutrients: Fat 61%;
Protein 19%; Carbs 20%

FOR THE BREAD
1 tablespoon coconut oil or butter, for greasing

1 (7-ounce) package cauliflower rice

2 eggs

6 tablespoons coconut flour

FOR THE FRENCH TOAST
¼ cup coconut or almond milk

1 teaspoon ground cinnamon

1 teaspoon nutmeg

2 tablespoons erythritol

1 egg

½ scoop Primal Kitchen Collagen Fuel Coconut-Vanilla
protein powder

½ teaspoon vanilla extract

2 tablespoons butter-flavored coconut oil or butter

½ cup sugar-free syrup (optional, but
highly recommended)

TO MAKE THE BREAD

1. Preheat the oven to 400°F. Grease a bread loaf pan with oil or butter.

2. In a bowl, combine the cauliflower rice, eggs, and flour and mix together.

3. Pour the mixture into the prepared loaf pan and bake for 15 to 20 minutes.

4. Remove the bread from the oven. Let cool in the pan for 20 to 30 minutes, then carefully remove from the pan (this bread is not going to rise), and cut into three equal pieces.

TO MAKE THE FRENCH TOAST

1. In a mixing bowl, combine the milk, cinnamon, nutmeg, erythritol, egg, protein powder, and vanilla and stir together.

2. Heat the coconut oil or butter in a shallow sauté pan over medium heat.

3. Carefully take a slice of the bread, dredge it in the milk mixture, and place it in the warm sauté pan. Repeat with the remaining 2 slices of bread.

4. Cook on one side for about 6 minutes (check to make sure it isn't burning—all cooktops are a bit different) and then carefully flip and cook on the other side for another 6 minutes or so.

5. Remove from the pan, transfer to plates, and drizzle sugar-free syrup over the top, if desired.

TIP: *You can find packages of pre-riced cauliflower in the freezer section of the grocery store; however, the brand I use for this recipe is called Fullgreen, which does not need to be refrigerated. I also highly recommend you make the bread in advance (a day or two even) because when it cools, it's far sturdier. If you want to make the bread for a use other than French toast, feel free to add herbs and spices of your choice to the mix in step 2 of the bread recipe.*

SWAP: *If you don't want to make the bread yourself, you can use keto-approved bread such as Julian Bakery brand and KNOW Foods, but making your own is really the best because you can control the ingredients.*

BREAKFAST SAUSAGE

PREP TIME: 5 MINUTES / COOK TIME: 10 TO 15 MINUTES

The problem with the majority of sausage products on the market is that they usually contain filler ingredients like sugar and nitrates. Reading ingredients labels is one approach you can take to make sure you're not consuming unhealthy ingredients, but you may wind up spending four hours at the grocery store each trip. Try something that takes far less time and never contains such ingredients: Make your own!

BULK COOK, ONE POT, SUPER QUICK

4
SERVINGS

Per Serving: Calories: 259; Total Fat: 19g; Total Carbohydrates: 2g; Net Carbs: 1g; Fiber: 1g; Protein: 20g

Macronutrients: Fat 66%; Protein 31%; Carbs 3%

TIP: *Make this recipe in bulk and you can add the sausage to salad greens on a different day.*

TRIVIA: *Fennel seeds contain antioxidants including kaempferol and quercetin, which have been linked to protection against infection, neurological diseases, and even cancer.*

1 pound ground meat (pork, beef, turkey, chicken, or bison)
2 teaspoons erythritol "brown sugar" or sugar-free maple syrup
1 tablespoon dried sage
1 tablespoon dried thyme
1 teaspoon fennel seeds
1 teaspoon salt
1 teaspoon red pepper flakes
1 teaspoon garlic powder
½ teaspoon paprika
½ teaspoon onion powder
1 tablespoon chopped fresh parsley (optional)
1 tablespoon butter, coconut oil, or avocado oil
1 fried egg, for serving (optional)
Spinach, sautéed, for serving (optional)

1. In a bowl, mix together the ground meat, erythritol, sage, thyme, fennel seeds, salt, red pepper flakes, garlic, paprika, onion powder, and parsley (if using) until well combined. Shape into 4 patties.

2. Heat the butter or oil in a sauté pan over medium-high heat.

3. Place the meat patties in the pan and cook about 5 minutes per side. (Depending on the type of meat you are using, the cook time could differ.)

4. Remove from the pan, transfer to plates, and serve with a fried egg and some sautéed spinach, if desired.

BREAKFAST BOWL WITH CAULIFLOWER HASH

PREP TIME: 10 MINUTES / COOK TIME: 15 TO 20 MINUTES

This is the heartiest bowl of satiating fat and protein that will fill you up for far longer than those Lucky Charms™ did. This meal is absolutely perfect if you plan on skipping your next meal (intermittent fasting), because it will tide you over for hours.

2 tablespoons avocado oil or butter, divided

3 tablespoons finely diced onion

½ cup riced or diced cauliflower

¼ tablespoon garlic powder, plus ½ teaspoon

Salt

Freshly ground black pepper

1 egg

½ cup peppers and onions (you can find this combination frozen at your grocery store)

¼ cup shredded cheese, plus more for serving (all optional)

½ cup raw spinach

1 serving Breakfast Sausage (page 58)

¼ cup minced tomatoes

Melted ghee or MCT oil, for serving (optional)

1. In a skillet, heat 1 tablespoon of avocado oil or butter over medium heat and evenly coat your pan.

2. Add the onion and let cook for about a minute. Add the cauliflower and cook for 3 minutes. Add ¼ tablespoon garlic powder, salt, and pepper and cook for 5 minutes more.

BREAKFAST BOWL WITH CAULIFLOWER HASH *continues*

SUPER QUICK

1
SERVING

Per Serving: Calories: 603; Total Fat: 47g; Total Carbohydrates: 16g; Net Carbs: 11g; Fiber: 5g; Protein: 29g

Macronutrients: Fat 70%; Protein 20%; Carbs 10%

TIP: *This is a great meal to make in advance and take with you on the go because it happens to be one of those recipes that is actually better as leftovers thanks to all of the flavors continuing to marinate together.*

SWAP: *If you're sick of cauliflower, you can use grated radish for the hash recipe.*

3. While the cauliflower hash is cooking, in another skillet, you can be cooking a sunny-side-up or over-easy egg and you can be heating up the peppers and onions with the remaining 1 tablespoon of avocado oil or butter, salt, pepper, and the remaining ½ teaspoon of garlic powder. If you want, you can scramble your egg with the peppers and onions.

4. Turn off the heat for the cauliflower and add the cheese (if using).

5. To construct the bowl, place the raw spinach at the bottom of the bowl, then add your cauliflower hash. Top that with the peppers and onions. Add the Breakfast Sausage and cooked egg, then sprinkle with the tomatoes and, if you'd like, top with cheese and drizzle with melted ghee or MCT oil.

COFFEE CAKE

PREP TIME: 5 TO 10 MINUTES / COOK TIME: 30 MINUTES

This recipe is not only delicious, but makes incorporating collagen into your diet easy. Collagen helps maintain the cartilage in our bodies—you know, the tissue that helps protect our joints from wear and tear. Plus, it's a piece of cake to make!

2 tablespoons coconut oil, divided

14 ounces brewed coffee (decaf or regular)

¾ cup coconut flour

1 cup protein powder of choice

1 scoop unflavored collagen

1 cup erythritol, plus more for serving (optional)

½ teaspoon vanilla extract

1 tablespoon ground cinnamon

4 eggs

Sugar-free maple syrup or Simple Ice Cream (page 181), for serving (optional)

1. Preheat the oven to 350°F. Grease an 8-inch square baking pan with 1 tablespoon of coconut oil.

2. In a blender, combine the remaining 1 tablespoon of coconut oil, coffee, coconut flour, protein powder, collagen, erythritol, vanilla, cinnamon, and eggs. Purée until fully combined and the batter has a pudding-like consistency.

3. Pour the contents of the blender into the prepared pan and bake for 30 minutes, or until the cake's texture is a cross between brownies and marshmallows (that's thanks to the collagen).

4. Remove the coffee cake from the oven and let cool for about 3 minutes before cutting into pieces. You can eat the cake as is, or sprinkle it with extra erythritol, drizzle it with some sugar-free syrup, or serve with a scoop of ice cream.

9-12
SERVINGS

Per Serving: Calories: 282; Total Fat: 10g; Total Carbohydrates: 20g; Net Carbs: 11g; Fiber: 11g; Protein: 28g; Erythritol Carbs: 21g

Macronutrients: Fat 32%; Protein 40%; Carbs 28%

TIP: *If you're craving that crumbly coffee-cake topping, combine ¼ cup of melted coconut oil, ½ cup of erythritol, and 1 teaspoon of ground cinnamon in a mixing bowl and drizzle over the top of your Coffee Cake.*

SWAP: *Feel free to use flavored protein or flavored collagen (chocolate or vanilla) for extra flavor. Also, if you have hit your protein allotment for the day (or plan on eating more protein later, swap in MCT oil powder for the collagen.*

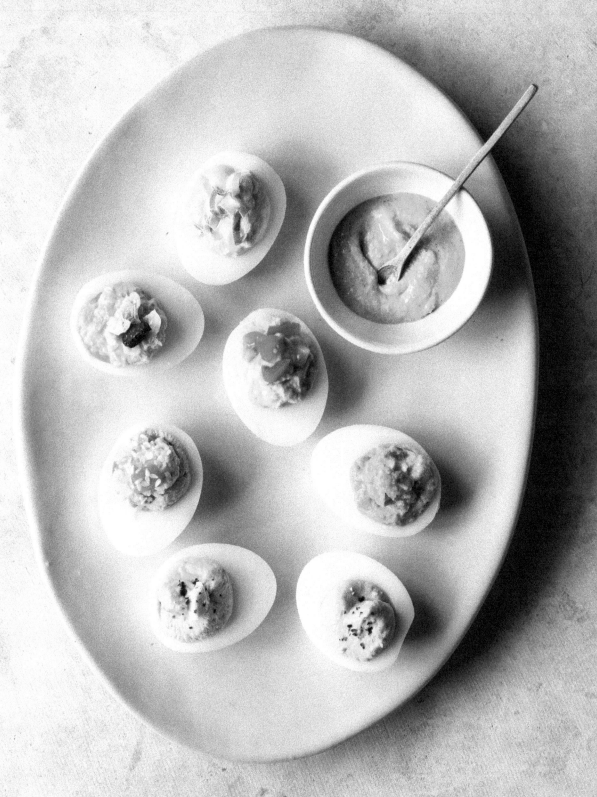

Deviled Eggs (7 Variations), page 64

Chapter 4

Sides & Snacks

Feeling peckish? Even though the keto diet will diminish your appetite, sometimes a snack is just necessary to tide you over until your next meal. These recipes are here to help you with that!

Deviled Eggs (7 Variations) **64**

Cauliflower Popcorn **67**

Pigs in a Blanket **68**

Sautéed Asparagus with Beef Jerky Sticks **70**

Scotch Eggs **71**

Eggplant Chips **72**

Asparagus Wrapped in Salmon Bacon **74**

Avocado Fries **75**

Nachos (3 Variations) **76**

Lemon–Poppy Seed Muffins **77**

DEVILED EGGS (7 VARIATIONS)

PREP TIME: 10 MINUTES / COOK TIME: 10 MINUTES

This twist on deviled eggs should not be called "deviled" at all because they aren't very spicy. If you're the type to add hot sauce to everything, then the name can stay. Otherwise, perhaps we should just call these stuffed eggs. Thankfully, though, this snack recipe will not stuff you because it's perfectly portioned and filling.

SUPER QUICK

1-2
SERVINGS

CLASSIC

Per Serving: Calories: 122;
Total Fat: 10g; Total
Carbohydrates: 1g; Net Carbs:
1g; Fiber: 0g; Protein: 7g

Macronutrients: Fat 74%;
Protein 23%; Carbs 3%

SARDINE OR SALMON

Per Serving: Calories: 179;
Total Fat: 11g; Total
Carbohydrates: 6g; Net Carbs:
4g; Fiber: 2g; Protein: 14g

Macronutrients: Fat 55%;
Protein 31% Carbs 14%

SPICY TUNA

Per Serving: Calories: 155;
Total Fat: 10g; Total
Carbohydrates: 1g; Net Carbs:
1g; Fiber: 0g; Protein: 15g

Macronutrients: Fat 60%;
Protein 37%; Carbs 3%

FOR ALL VARIATIONS
2 eggs

FOR CLASSIC VARIATION
1 egg yolk
2 tablespoons minced scallions
½ teaspoon spicy mustard
½ tablespoon olive or avocado oil
1 teaspoon salt
1 teaspoon freshly ground black pepper

1. Bring a small pot of water to a boil on the stove. Place the eggs in the water using a slotted spoon. Cook for about 10 minutes.

2. Meanwhile, prepare an ice bath for the eggs by filling a bowl with water and ice.

3. While the eggs are cooking, prep specific ingredients depending on which variety of deviled egg you'd like to make.

4. When the eggs are finished, use a slotted spoon to remove them from the pot and transfer to the ice bath to cool.

5. When the eggs are cool, carefully peel them (the ice bath should have helped them peel easier). Slice them in half lengthwise. Scoop out the egg yolks, without harming the egg whites, and put them in a mixing bowl.

6. Add the specific ingredients for the variation you're making to the bowl and mix together well.

7. Using a small spoon, fill each egg white cavity with the mixture and devour!

OTHER POSSIBLE VARIATIONS

FOR SARDINE OR SALMON VARIATION

1 egg yolk

½ can sardines or salmon, packed in water or olive oil

2 cherry tomatoes, diced

¼ small avocado, mashed (if using sardines or salmon packed in water)

½ teaspoon mustard

FOR SPICY TUNA VARIATION

1 egg yolk

2 ounces sushi-grade ahi tuna

½ teaspoon sesame oil

½ teaspoon spicy mustard

1 teaspoon tamari or coconut aminos

Sesame seeds, for garnish

FOR GROUND BEEF VARIATION

1 egg yolk

2 ounces ground beef

¼ small avocado, mashed

Salt

Freshly ground black pepper

FOR CHICKEN VARIATION

1 egg yolk

2 ounces ground or diced chicken (thigh or breast, depending on preference)

2 teaspoons diced tomatoes

¼ small avocado, mashed, or ½ tablespoon olive or avocado oil

1 teaspoon garlic powder

1 teaspoon onion powder

Salt

Freshly ground black pepper

Sugar-free hot sauce (optional)

GROUND BEEF

Per Serving: Calories: 248; Total Fat: 16g; Total Carbohydrates: 3g; Net Carbs: 1g; Fiber: 2g; Protein: 13g

Macronutrients: Fat 60%; Protein 37%; Carbs 3%

CHICKEN

Per Serving: Calories: 180; Total Fat: 12g; Total Carbohydrates: 3g; Net Carbs: 2g; Fiber: 1g; Protein: 15g

Macronutrients: Fat 60%; Protein 33%; Carbs 7%

MEXICAN-STYLE

Per Serving: Calories: 147; Total Fat: 11g; Total Carbohydrates: 4g; Net Carbs: 2g; Fiber: 2g; Protein: 8g

Macronutrients: Fat 68%; Protein 22%; Carbs 10%

THANKSGIVING-STYLE

Per Serving: Calories: 149; Total Fat: 9g; Total Carbohydrates: 2g; Net Carbs: 1g; Fiber: 1g; Protein: 15g

Macronutrients: Fat 54%; Protein 40%; Carbs 6%

DEVILED EGGS (7 VARIATIONS) *continues*

TIP: You can find pre-roasted Brussels sprouts at places like Trader Joe's. Mashed or puréed pumpkin and butternut squash can be found in cans in the canned vegetable aisle. You can also pur-chase premade diced or shredded chicken and turkey from the salad bar at your local grocery store.

SWAP: *Feel free to use avocado oil mayon-naise (plain, chipotle lime, garlic aioli) instead of olive oil or avocado for any of these deviled egg variations. You can also top with or mix in sugar-free hot sauce for any of them.*

FOR MEXICAN-STYLE VARIATION

1 egg yolk

¼ small avocado, mashed

1 tablespoon salsa (mild, medium, or hot depending on preference)

Salt

Freshly ground black pepper

FOR THANKSGIVING-STYLE VARIATION

1 egg yolk

2 tablespoons mashed or puréed pumpkin or butternut squash

2 tablespoons diced Roasted Brussels Sprouts (page 108)

2 ounces diced turkey (thigh or breast, depending on preference)

1 or 2 sugar-free fresh cranberries, for topping (optional)

CAULIFLOWER POPCORN

PREP TIME: 5 MINUTES / COOK TIME: 40 MINUTES

Popcorn is one of those foods that some believe is healthy and others don't. Contrary to popular belief, corn is not a vegetable—it's a high-carbohydrate grain, which means that from a keto perspective, it falls into the unhealthy category. This "popcorn" recipe uses vitamin C–rich cauliflower as a substitute for the beloved crunchy snack, so you can chomp away without the guilt.

Nonstick avocado oil cooking spray, for greasing

1 small to medium head cauliflower, florets with stems chopped into bite-size pieces

½ cup avocado oil

½ cup neutral-flavored grass-fed/-finished collagen protein powder (optional)

Popcorn seasonings of choice: salt, freshly ground black pepper, garlic powder, onion powder, dried oregano, dried sage, and/or nutritional yeast

1. Preheat the oven to 400°F. Coat a broiling pan with nonstick avocado oil spray. (If you have an air fryer, you can make your Cauliflower Popcorn in there instead; just coat the fryer basket with nonstick spray.)

2. Put the cauliflower in a mixing bowl. Pour the avocado oil over the top and sprinkle in the protein powder. Add the seasonings of your choice to the bowl. Stir all together to evenly coat the cauliflower.

3. Spread the cauliflower in an even layer on the prepared pan and place in the oven (or pour into your air fryer). Cook for roughly 40 minutes, checking periodically and stirring every 10 minutes or so (same goes for the air fryer, if using).

4. Remove from the oven (or air fryer) and serve.

BULK COOK, ONE POT

2-3
SERVINGS

Per Serving: Calories: 389; Total Fat: 37g; Total Carbohydrates: 10g; Net Carbs: 5g; Fiber: 5g; Protein: 4g

Macronutrients: Fat 86%; Protein 4%; Carbs 10%

SWAP: *Craving kettle corn? Nix the savory seasonings and instead sprinkle with erythritol, powdered monk fruit extract, and/or sugar-free syrup. You may also want to use coconut oil as opposed to avocado oil to give the recipe even more sweetness.*

PIGS IN A BLANKET

PREP TIME: 5 MINUTES / COOK TIME: 15 MINUTES

When I was a kid, I remember snatching more than my fair share of those premade pigs in a blanket whenever I went to family functions. It was heaven to be ignorant of the contents of these little piggies, which are certainly not keto-friendly. Fret not, though. Thanks to this easy modified recipe, you don't have to rid your life—or your parties—of pigs in a blanket.

**ONE POT,
SUPER QUICK**

2-4
SERVINGS

Per Serving: Calories: 265;
Total Fat: 22g; Total
Carbohydrates: 11g; Net Carbs:
5g; Fiber: 6g; Protein: 9g

Macronutrients: Fat 72%;
Protein 13%; Carbs 15%

2 tablespoons avocado oil, divided
1 small eggplant
Salt
1 tablespoon oregano
Freshly ground black pepper
2 precooked beef or chicken hot dogs (must be sugar-free)
Sugar-free ketchup and/or mustard, for serving

1. Preheat the oven to 400°F. Grease a baking sheet with 1 tablespoon of avocado oil.

2. Slice the eggplant lengthwise, lay on the baking sheet, and sprinkle with salt. Let sit for 3 to 4 minutes to let the moisture come to the surface. Get a damp towel and wipe the salt off the eggplant slices.

3. Brush the eggplant with the remaining 1 tablespoon of avocado oil, then sprinkle with the oregano and pepper.

4. Roast the eggplant for about 10 minutes, flipping halfway through cooking.

5. Remove the eggplant from the oven and let cool for a few minutes. While the eggplant is cooling, cut each hot dog into three equal pieces.

6. Slice each piece of eggplant lengthwise into two or three "sheets," then wrap one sheet snugly around each piece of hot dog.

7. Transfer the wrapped hot dogs to the baking sheet and roast for 5 minutes.

8. Remove from the oven, place a toothpick in each pig in a blanket, and serve with ketchup and/or mustard!

TIP: *Don't want to go through the hassle of preparing eggplant? You may be able to find it premade in the prepared food section of your grocery store, but do ask what ingredients were used while cooking, because sometimes unnecessary ingredients are added.*

SWAP: *Feel free to use pork hot dogs in this recipe, but make sure they're 100 percent sugar-free and contain no nitrates. Also, if you're not an eggplant fan, you can use grilled or broiled zucchini.*

BRAND: *The grass-fed and -finished beef hot dog brands I recommend are Teton Waters Ranch or Applegate Farms. As for chicken hot dogs, I recommend the brand Bilinski's.*

SAUTÉED ASPARAGUS WITH BEEF JERKY STICKS

PREP TIME: 5 MINUTES / COOK TIME: 10 TO 15 MINUTES

One Christmas my mom bought me 20 bags of beef jerky as a gift. I ate them all, as one does, straight out of the bag in less than a week. Even if you don't love beef jerky or beef sticks as much as I do, these items can be great as ingredients in actual dishes (not just as snacks), as you'll see with this recipe.

ONE POT, SUPER QUICK

1
SERVING

Per Serving: Calories: 665; Total Fat: 64g; Total Carbohydrates: 9g; Net Carbs: 6g; Fiber: 3g; Protein: 16g

Macronutrients: Fat 86%; Protein 9%; Carbs 5%

BRAND: *The beef sticks I have always used for this recipe are Chomps; however, there are lots of meat stick brands on the market these days that are amazing, such as Nick's Sticks and Paleovalley. Just make sure they're sugar-free.*

5 tablespoons olive oil

10 asparagus spears, trimmed

2 beef jerky sticks, diced

¾ teaspoon garlic powder

Salt

Freshly ground black pepper

1 fried egg, for serving (optional)

1. Pour the olive oil into a sauté pan and place over medium-high heat. Add the asparagus and cook for 5 to 6 minutes, stirring occasionally.

2. Add the jerky, garlic powder, salt, and pepper and stir. Cover and cook for another few minutes, depending on how you like your asparagus.

3. Serve this with a fried egg if you'd like for a little extra fat and protein.

TIP: *If fresh asparagus is too expensive, venture into the freezer section and grab a bag or two of the frozen variety.*

SWAP: *You can use beef jerky instead of beef sticks in this recipe if you so choose. Grass-Fed Jerky Chews from Sophia's Survival Food are a great option; just take into account that macronutrients could change slightly.*

SCOTCH EGGS

PREP TIME: 10 MINUTES / COOK TIME: 25 MINUTES

What came first, the chicken or the egg? Well, in this case, the chicken is nowhere in sight, so the brain-boosting (thanks to its amazing supply of choline) egg comes first, because you need to boil it up and then wrap the ground meat around it!

1 tablespoon coconut oil

1 egg

¼ pound ground beef (80 percent lean)

1 teaspoon garlic powder

1 teaspoon onion powder

¼ teaspoon ground sumac

¼ teaspoon salt

¼ teaspoon freshly ground black pepper

¼ teaspoon ground saffron

Olive oil, for drizzling

1. Preheat the oven to 350°F. Line a baking sheet with aluminum foil and coat with the coconut oil.

2. Bring a small pot of water to a boil. Place the egg in the water using a slotted spoon. Cook for about 10 minutes.

3. Meanwhile, in a bowl, combine the beef with the garlic, onion, sumac, salt, pepper, and saffron and mix together.

4. When the egg is done cooking, use a slotted spoon to transfer it to an ice bath or the fridge to cool. Once cool enough to handle, peel the egg.

5. Wrap the meat mixture around the egg, making sure to cover it entirely. Place on the prepared baking sheet and bake for 10 to 15 minutes.

6. Take out of the oven, let cool, and enjoy with a little drizzle of olive oil.

1
SERVING

Per Serving: Calories: 468; Total Fat: 40g; Total Carbohydrates: 2g; Net Carbs: 2g; Fiber: 0g; Protein: 25g

Macronutrients: Fat 77%; Protein 21%; Carbs 2%

TIP: *If you don't want to buy all of these spices individually, try to find kebab seasoning in the spice aisle at the grocery store.*

SWAP: *If you're in a crunch for time, feel free to use premade hard-boiled eggs, which can be found in the deli section at the grocery store.*

EGGPLANT CHIPS

PREP TIME: 10 MINUTES / COOK TIME: 35 MINUTES

You probably won't be surprised to hear that chips are the most popular snack food in America. While you'll want to avoid the potato variety, you can still eat various types of chips on keto, including this delightful recipe. One day, maybe you'll even find bags of this recipe in the chip aisle. It certainly satisfies the urge for some crunch!

BULK COOK

2
SERVINGS

Per Serving: Calories: 270; Total Fat: 22g; Total Carbohydrates: 15g; Net Carbs: 6g; Fiber: 9g; Protein: 3g

Macronutrients: Fat 73%; Protein 5%; Carbs 22%

3 tablespoons olive oil, divided

1 medium eggplant, sliced into ½-inch-thick rounds

2 teaspoons salt

1 teaspoon garlic powder, plus more if desired

1 teaspoon dried oregano, plus more if desired

½ teaspoon freshly ground black pepper, plus more if desired

Guacamole (page 210), Bean-Free Hummus (page 211), or Butternut Squash "Cheese" Sauce (page 216), for serving (optional)

1. Preheat the oven to 350°F. Line a baking sheet with foil and grease with 1 tablespoon of the olive oil.

2. Sprinkle the eggplant slices with the salt. Let sit for 3 to 4 minutes to let the moisture come to the surface. Get a damp towel and wipe the salt off the eggplant slices.

3. Pour the remaining 2 tablespoons of olive oil into a bowl. Lay the eggplant slices on the prepared baking sheet and, using a food brush, "paint" them with the olive oil. Sprinkle with the garlic powder, oregano, and pepper.

4. Bake the eggplant chips for 35 minutes, or until they're browned, flipping halfway through cooking and painting the other side with the olive oil. Feel free to sprinkle more garlic powder, oregano, and pepper on top if you'd like.

5. Remove the eggplant chips from the oven and let cool.

6. Serve with Guacamole, Bean-Free Hummus, or Butternut Squash "Cheese" Sauce, if desired.

TIP: *Do not venture too far from your kitchen when you make these chips, because you want to check on them periodically to make sure they don't burn. You can also broil the chips for two to three minutes at the end of the cooking time to make them crispier.*

SWAP: *You can easily swap out the eggplant for zucchini or summer squash, but the baking time might change slightly. Another way to cook these chips perfectly is with an air fryer.*

ASPARAGUS WRAPPED IN SALMON BACON

PREP TIME: 5 MINUTES / COOK TIME: 25 TO 30 MINUTES

I adore my husband, but even he knows that my true love is salmon bacon. I even told him in my wedding vows that salmon comes first, and he comes second, which he was okay with. Clearly my obsession is real, and when you taste omega-3-rich salmon bacon, you might be listing your significant other second, as well.

BULK COOK, ONE POT

2
SERVINGS

Per Serving: Calories: 319; Total Fat: 23g; Total Carbohydrates: 5g; Net Carbs: 2g; Fiber: 3g; Protein: 23g

Macronutrients: Fat 65%; Protein 29%; Carbs 6%

SWAP: *If you don't want to deal with trying to find salmon skin, you can thinly slice a salmon fillet instead.*

TRIVIA: *You may have never heard of salmon bacon before, but you might already be eating it unknowingly. It's actually salmon belly, which is the thinnest part of a fillet.*

Coconut oil, for greasing and drizzling
8 ounces skin-on salmon belly, cut into 5-by-5-inch squares
8 jumbo asparagus spears, trimmed

1. Preheat the oven to broil. Coat a baking sheet with coconut oil.

2. In a shallow pot over medium-high heat, bring 3 cups of water to a boil. Add the asparagus and cook for about 3 minutes. Remove from the pot immediately and submerge in ice water or place in the refrigerator for a few minutes.

3. Take asparagus out of the ice water or refrigerator and wrap a piece of salmon skin/belly, flesh-side up, tightly around each spear.

4. Transfer the wrapped asparagus to the prepared baking sheet and broil for 20 to 25 minutes. Halfway through the broiling time, use tongs to carefully flip the wrapped asparagus.

5. To serve, drizzle a little coconut oil over the wrapped asparagus.

TIP: *Short on time? Wrap smoked salmon around lightly steamed asparagus instead.*

AVOCADO FRIES

PREP TIME: 10 MINUTES / COOK TIME: 15 TO 20 MINUTES

I am pretty sure the sensational texture combination of crispy and creamy is everyone's fantasy. Well, this monounsaturated-fat-laden recipe will make that divine combo a reality!

Avocado oil, coconut oil, or butter, for greasing

1 egg

1 teaspoon lime juice, plus more for serving (all optional)

¼ cup almond flour

2 tablespoons flax meal

1 avocado, halved, pitted, peeled, and sliced into strips

Sea salt, chipotle powder, or sugar-free hot sauce, for serving (optional)

1. Preheat the oven to 450°F. Line a baking sheet with aluminum foil and grease with oil or butter. (Alternatively, you can use an air fryer—no need to preheat anything, but you will need to grease the fryer basket.)

2. In a shallow mixing bowl, whisk the egg and lime juice (if using).

3. In another shallow mixing bowl, mix together the almond flour and flax meal.

4. Carefully dip each avocado strip in the egg wash and then in the flour mixture. Set on the prepared baking sheet (or put in an air fryer).

5. Bake the avocado strips for about 20 minutes (or air-fry for about 15 minutes), or until crisp, flipping them halfway through cooking.

6. Serve your fries with an extra squeeze of lime juice and a sprinkle of sea salt, or add a little extra spiciness by sprinkling them with chipotle powder or drizzling some hot sauce on top!

SUPER QUICK

2
SERVINGS

Per Serving: Calories: 252; Total Fat: 20g; Total Carbohydrates: 11g; Net Carbs: 3g; Fiber: 8g; Protein: 7g

Macronutrients: Fat 71%; Protein 11%; Carbs 18%

SWAP: *I have made this recipe both with almond flour and with coconut flour. If you can eat nuts, stick with almond flour, as it seems to create a better crunch.*

TRIVIA: *Did you know that avocados have more potassium than bananas?*

NACHOS (3 VARIATIONS)

PREP TIME: 10 MINUTES / COOK TIME: 35 MINUTES

These are na-cho average nachos! This recipe emphasizes the use of grass-fed/-finished dairy, which supplies omega-3 fats, making it a guilt-free crunch-fest. Speaking of crunch, let's be real: Nachos are not nachos without that crisp snap of the chip, and thankfully Eggplant Chips (page 72) will give you just that.

2
SERVINGS

Per Serving: Calories: 833;
Total Fat: 73g; Total
Carbohydrates: 21g; Net Carbs:
11g; Fiber: 10g; Protein: 33g

Macronutrients: Fat 79%;
Protein 16%; Carbs 5%

OTHER POSSIBLE VARIATIONS

FOR THE VEGAN CHEESE SAUCE VARIATION
1 recipe Butternut Squash "Cheese" Sauce (page 216)

FOR THE MELTED CHEESE VARIATION
1 tablespoon butter or coconut butter

8 ounces grass-fed/-finished Cheddar or pepper Jack cheese

FOR ALL VARIATIONS
1 recipe Eggplant Chips (page 72)

Sliced scallions, for garnish

FOR THE CHEESE SAUCE VARIATION
2 tablespoons butter

½ cup grass-fed/-finished whole milk

1 teaspoon garlic powder

½ teaspoon onion powder

½ teaspoon paprika

8 ounces grass-fed/-finished Cheddar cheese

1. Put the Eggplant Chips on a plate.
2. If you're making the cheese sauce, melt the butter in a skillet over medium heat. Add the milk, garlic powder, onion powder, and paprika and stir. Remove the mixture from the heat, add the cheese, and stir until melted.
3. If you're making the melted cheese variation, melt the butter in a sauté pan, then add the cheese, turn the heat to low, and gently stir until the cheese is completely melted.
4. Pour the cheese sauce or Butternut Squash "Cheese" Sauce over the Eggplant Chips (you may need to use a spoon to help you with this), and garnish with scallions.

TIP: *If you want to make this into a more substantial meal, add crumbled ground beef, pork, turkey, or chicken to the Nachos.*

LEMON–POPPY SEED MUFFINS

PREP TIME: 10 MINUTES / COOK TIME: 20 TO 25 MINUTES

When my sister learned to drive, a Pandora's box of food opened for us both. Our favorite "sweet ride" was going to the local bakery to buy lemon–poppy seed muffins. Luckily, I have replicated the recipe in keto fashion, so I can keep eating them—and so can you!

¼ cup coconut flour

¼ cup coconut oil, melted

2 eggs

¼ cup erythritol

2 tablespoons freshly squeezed lemon juice

1 teaspoon lemon zest (optional)

½ teaspoon baking powder

Pinch salt

1½ tablespoons poppy seeds

1 tablespoon collagen powder

½ teaspoon vanilla extract

MCT oil or butter-flavored coconut oil (optional)

1. Preheat the oven to 350°F. Line a muffin tin with muffin cup liners.

2. In a mixing bowl, combine the coconut flour, coconut oil, eggs, erythritol, lemon juice, lemon zest (if using), baking powder, salt, poppy seeds, collagen powder, and vanilla and mix until smooth.

3. Divide the batter among the muffin cups and bake for 20 to 25 minutes.

4. Turn off the oven. Let the muffins cool in the oven for about 20 minutes.

5. To serve, drizzle with MCT oil, if you'd like, or you can use Barlean's flavored fish or flax oils.

BULK COOK

3
SERVINGS

Per Serving: Calories: 325; Total Fat: 25g; Total Carbohydrates: 15g; Net Carbs: 6g; Fiber: 9g; Protein: 10g; Erythritol Carbs: 18g

Macronutrients: Fat 70%; Protein 12%; Carbs 18%

TIP: *If you don't have a muffin tin, you can use a loaf pan.*

SWAP: *If you cannot consume eggs, you can use "flax eggs" instead. To make these faux eggs, combine 2 tablespoons of ground flaxseeds and 6 tablespoons of water.*

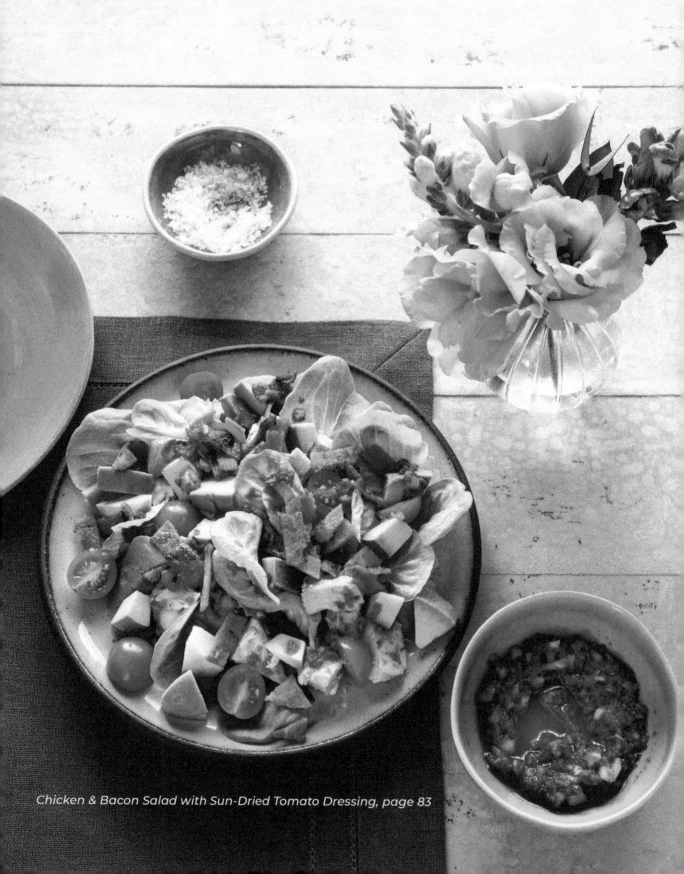

Chicken & Bacon Salad with Sun-Dried Tomato Dressing, page 83

Chapter 5

Soups & Salads

"Lettuce" celebrate the fact that these recipes are "souper" because they incorporate low-carbohydrate vegetables—you can eat a lot of them without going over your daily carbohydrate threshold!

Niçoise Salad 80

Leek & Cauliflower Soup 82

Chicken & Bacon Salad with Sun-Dried Tomato Dressing 83

Basic Chicken Salad in Lettuce Cups 85

Chicken Soup 86

Roasted Vegetable Salad 87

Chopped Bitter Greens Salad 89

Minestrone Soup 90

Cobb Salad 92

Asian Cucumber Salad 94

Cauliflower "Potato" Salad 95

Lobster BLT Salad 96

NIÇOISE SALAD

PREP TIME: 15 MINUTES / COOK TIME: 45 MINUTES

Each ingredient in this salad has its own personality, so it's great for entertaining guests because you can mix and match ingredients to please everyone's palate. You can even plate each ingredient individually and let people choose their own combination of base, protein, toppings, sauces, and sides.

2
SERVINGS

Per Serving: Calories: 738; Total Fat: 58g; Total Carbohydrates: 15g; Net Carbs: 8g; Fiber: 7g; Protein: 39g

Macronutrients: Fat 71%; Protein 21%; Carbs 8%

1 head kohlrabi, peeled and cut into cubes
2 tablespoons avocado oil, divided
1 cup fresh or frozen green beans
8 ounces sushi-grade ahi tuna steak
2 eggs
1 (8-ounce) bag butter lettuce
½ pint cherry tomatoes, halved
6 anchovy fillets (optional)
3 tablespoons capers
3 tablespoons Niçoise olives
5 tablespoons olive oil
2 tablespoons white wine vinegar
3 tablespoons Dijon mustard
Salt
Freshly ground black pepper

1. Preheat the oven to 450°F. Line a baking sheet with aluminum foil.

2. Spread the kohlrabi out evenly on the baking sheet. Coat with 1 tablespoon of avocado oil, then roast for about 45 minutes, tossing occasionally.

3. Meanwhile, fill a pot with ¼ cup of water, add the green beans, and steam for 8 to 10 minutes (if using frozen, steam in the microwave on high power for 5 to 8 minutes).

4. When there are 15 minutes of cook time left for the kohlrabi, heat the remaining 1 tablespoon of avocado oil in a shallow skillet over medium-high heat. Add the tuna and sear to your desired doneness, 2 to 3 minutes per side for rare.

5. While the tuna is searing, prepare the eggs any way you'd like them: poached, sunny-side up, over easy, hard- or soft-boiled.

6. Slice the tuna into two equal pieces. Lay butter lettuce on each of two plates. Top with the tuna, eggs, green beans, tomatoes, anchovies (if using), capers, and olives.

7. In a bowl, combine the olive oil, vinegar, mustard, salt, and pepper and whisk until smooth and creamy. Drizzle the dressing over the salad and enjoy!

TIP: *If you want meals for days, you can easily quadruple this recipe. All of the ingredients keep well in the fridge for a few days (though be mindful of the fish!), so this salad is perfect to bring to work.*

SWAP: *Feel free to use canned tuna (or salmon, sardines, or mackerel) if you wish; just make sure the fish is packed in olive oil. You can use the oil as extra dressing for your salad. You can also use grilled salmon instead of the ahi tuna.*

LEEK & CAULIFLOWER SOUP

PREP TIME: 10 MINUTES / COOK TIME: 30 TO 45 MINUTES

I've made this recipe several times, with ingredients purchased from your run-of-the-mill grocery store and from vendors at farmers' markets. Every time I have made it with the vegetables from local vendors, I can taste a difference! So use fresh produce for this recipe and you won't regret it.

4

SERVINGS

Per Serving: Calories: 266; Total Fat: 18g; Total Carbohydrates: 17g; Net Carbs: 11g; Fiber: 5g; Protein: 9g

Macronutrients: Fat 61%; Protein 14%; Carbs 25%

TRIVIA: *Rutabaga is a root vegetable, which generally tend not to be so keto-friendly. However, if you balance your macros correctly, you can include it here and there! Rutabaga is low in calories and has roughly 7 net carbs per 3.5 ounces.*

2 tablespoons olive oil

3 leeks, cleaned, white and light green parts sliced into rounds

1 head cauliflower, coarsely chopped

¼ rutabaga, peeled and cut into cubes

2 garlic cloves, minced

1 (32-ounce) container vegetable broth

½ cup full-fat coconut milk

Paprika, for serving (optional)

Chopped fresh basil or oregano, for serving (optional)

Parsley sprigs, for serving

1. Heat the olive oil in a large pot over medium-high heat.
2. Add the leeks, cauliflower, rutabaga, and garlic to the pot and sauté for about 5 minutes.
3. Pour the vegetable broth and coconut milk into the pot, cover, and cook for 30 minutes.
4. Transfer the contents of the pot to a blender or food processor and blend until the soup achieves a liquid yogurt-like consistency.
5. Let the soup cool, transfer to bowls, and sprinkle with paprika, basil, or oregano, if you'd like. Serve with sprigs of parsley on top.

SWAP: *Ditch the rutabaga if you don't want the extra carbohydrates. You can also throw in some diced chicken to make this a complete meal.*

CHICKEN & BACON SALAD WITH SUN-DRIED TOMATO DRESSING

PREP TIME: 10 MINUTES / COOK TIME: 5 MINUTES

I guess you could call this salad a BLT of sorts, with some chicken added—so maybe it's a BLTC. I call it a BLT for a completely different reason, though. You see, over the years I have known my friend Brittany, she went from being a strict vegan to a bacon fiend. As Brittany is one of my all-time favorite women, she inspired me to create this BLT salad; BLT stands for Brittany's Loaded Tossed (Salad).

2 slices bacon

3 sun-dried tomatoes (packed in olive oil)

1 tablespoon olive oil

1 teaspoon minced shallots

¼ teaspoon garlic powder

½ teaspoon dried oregano

1 teaspoon nutritional yeast or grated cheese (optional but recommended)

½ teaspoon freshly squeezed lemon juice (optional)

Pinch each salt and freshly ground black pepper

1 cup Bibb or butter lettuce leaves

4 ounces cooked chicken breast and/or thigh meat, diced (if you use store-bought, make sure it doesn't contain any added sugar)

¼ cup cherry tomatoes, halved

½ avocado, pitted, peeled, and diced

SUPER QUICK

1

SERVING

Per Serving: Calories: 858; Total Fat: 62g; Total Carbohydrates: 23g; Net Carbs: 9g; Fiber: 14g; Protein: 52g

Macronutrients: Fat 65%; Protein 24%; Carbs 11%

CHICKEN & BACON SALAD WITH SUN-DRIED TOMATO DRESSING *continues*

SWAP: *If you don't want to make the dressing but still want the sun-dried tomato taste, you can use the sun-dried tomatoes in place of the cherry tomatoes and drizzle the olive oil that the tomatoes are packed in over the top of the salad.*

1. Heat a shallow skillet over medium heat. When warm, cook the bacon to your desired crispness, about 5 minutes. Turn off the heat and let the bacon sit in the skillet.

2. To make the dressing, in a blender, combine the sun-dried tomatoes, olive oil, shallots, garlic powder, oregano, nutritional yeast or cheese (if using), lemon juice (if using), and salt and pepper. Whirl away until smooth.

3. To construct the salad, put the lettuce on a plate. Top with the chicken, cherry tomatoes, and avocado. Lay the bacon on top (alternatively, you can chop up the bacon and sprinkle it on after you've dressed the salad). If you'd like, pour the bacon pan drippings over the salad (trust me, it's amazing). Spoon on about 1 to 2 tablespoons of dressing and dig in!

TIP: *Some brands of sun-dried tomatoes are packed in olive oil and include herbs and spices, which can certainly jazz up the dressing even more.*

BASIC CHICKEN SALAD IN LETTUCE CUPS

PREP TIME: 10 MINUTES

Chicken salad doesn't always get the best rap because it's typically made with omega-6-laden mayonnaise. That said, this jazzed-up recipe is studded with colorful antioxidant-packed gems and made with mayonnaise that you can feel good about eating, thanks to the healthy avocado oil it's made with.

8 ounces cooked chicken breast, diced (if using store-bought, make sure it's sugar-free)

½ red bell pepper, diced

¼ cup diced jicama

1 celery stalk, diced

2 tablespoons Primal Kitchen avocado oil mayonnaise

1 teaspoon Dijon mustard

4 slices cooked bacon, chopped

Splash freshly squeezed lemon juice

1 teaspoon fresh dill

Salt

Freshly ground black pepper

4 romaine or butter lettuce leaves

1 tablespoon sliced almonds (optional)

Chopped fresh parsley, for serving (optional)

1. In a mixing bowl, toss together the chicken, bell pepper, jicama, and celery.

2. Add the mayonnaise, mustard, bacon, and lemon juice, then sprinkle in the dill, season with salt and pepper, and stir everything together.

3. Arrange the lettuce leaves on plates and scoop in the chicken salad mixture.

4. Sprinkling almonds and parsley on top before serving is completely optional but gives these cups a little extra flavor and a nutritional boost!

QUICK

2
SERVINGS

Per Serving: Calories: 454; Total Fat: 30g; Total Carbohydrates: 8g; Net Carbs: 6g; Fiber: 2g; Protein: 36g

Macronutrients: Fat 61%; Protein 32%; Carbs 7%

SWAP: *Feel free to swap in cashews, macadamia nuts, or walnuts, though macronutrients may vary.*

BRAND: *There are so many different mayonnaise flavors these days. You can use plain, garlic, or a spicy variety for this recipe. If you don't eat eggs, the Primal Kitchen brand also makes an egg-free mayonnaise.*

CHICKEN SOUP

PREP TIME: 15 MINUTES / COOK TIME: 45 MINUTES

When I was younger and living with my parents, my mom used to make me this chicken soup when I got sick. It seemed to cure all of my ailments, and, as a bonus, it was delicious. I certainly hope it will do the same for you, or at least cure you of wondering what to make for lunch or dinner!

BULK COOK, ONE POT

4
SERVINGS

Per Serving: Calories: 323;
Total Fat: 19g; Total
Carbohydrates: 10g;
Net Carbs: 7g; Fiber: 3g;
Protein: 28g

Macronutrients: Fat 53%;
Protein 35%; Carbs 12%

TRIVIA: *Basil and garlic have actually been shown to be antimicrobial and antibacterial, which means they could potentially aid in soothing stomachaches and other digestive distress. The sodium in the broth can help replenish electrolytes that may have been lost during illness.*

3 tablespoons olive oil

1 (14-ounce) bag frozen peppers and onions

1 pound chicken thigh meat, diced

1 tablespoon dried thyme

½ tablespoon garlic powder

1 teaspoon salt

1 teaspoon freshly ground black pepper

1 (32-ounce) container chicken or vegetable broth, or Bone Broth (page 203)

½ pound spinach

1 teaspoon dried basil (optional)

1. Heat the oil in a large pot over medium heat.

2. Add the peppers and onions and cook until no longer frozen, 8 to 10 minutes.

3. Add the chicken and cook, stirring occasionally.

4. Stir in the thyme, garlic powder, salt, and pepper. Add the broth and cook for about 25 minutes.

5. Add the spinach and cook for another 5 minutes.

6. Serve the soup in bowls, sprinkled with the basil (if using).

SWAP: *Feel free to use turkey in this recipe instead of chicken. You can also add tomatoes.*

ROASTED VEGETABLE SALAD

PREP TIME: 15 MINUTES / COOK TIME: 45 MINUTES

I'm the type of person who loves the toppings in a salad more than the leafy greens. When I go to salad bars to feast, my salads are typically spilling off my plate because I load up on accompaniments. This salad makes the supporting vegetables the stars of the dish.

½ eggplant, diced

1 medium bulb fennel, diced

12 asparagus spears, diced

1 zucchini, diced

12 Brussels sprouts, halved

1 cup cubed fresh pumpkin

1 medium red or white onion, diced

4 tablespoons avocado oil

1 teaspoon minced garlic or garlic powder

1 teaspoon dried oregano or marjoram (or both)

1 teaspoon dried thyme

Salt

Freshly ground black pepper

2 cups mixed greens (or any salad greens of choice)

Freshly grated Parmesan cheese, for serving (optional)

16 ounces steak or black cod, for serving (optional)

4

SERVINGS

Per Serving: Calories: 227; Total Fat: 15g; Total Carbohydrates: 19g; Net Carbs: 12g; Fiber: 7g; Protein: 4g

Macronutrients: Fat 60%; Protein 8%; Carbs 32%

1. Preheat the oven to 450°F.

2. In a mixing bowl, combine the eggplant, fennel, asparagus, zucchini, Brussels sprouts, pumpkin, and onion. Pour in the avocado oil, add the garlic, oregano or marjoram, and thyme, and season with salt and pepper. Mix together until the vegetables are well coated.

ROASTED VEGETABLE SALAD *continues*

SWAP: *You can use coconut oil instead of avocado oil for an even sweeter flavor. Or you can use butter.*

TRIVIA: *Not only is this recipe bursting with flavor, but it's also bursting with B vitamins, iron, and folate, which are extremely female-friendly.*

3. Spread the vegetables in an even layer on a baking sheet and roast for 35 to 45 minutes, checking occasionally and stirring every 15 to 20 minutes. (Your oven may be very powerful, so feel free to take the veggies out sooner than 35 minutes if they are browned to your liking.)

4. Divide the greens among four plates and evenly distribute the roasted vegetables on top. Sprinkle with freshly grated cheese and serve with steak or cod, if desired.

TIP: *Instead of roasting all these vegetables yourself, you can purchase them pre-grilled in the freezer section of Trader Joe's or in the prepared food section of your grocery store. Just be sure to read the ingredients before buying.*

CHOPPED BITTER GREENS SALAD

PREP TIME: 10 MINUTES

My mother is not a bitter person, but her palate is! She loves a bitter flavor, so she is the inspiration for this salad because she makes a huge bowl of it every single night with dinner. Every. Single. Night.

1 ounce arugula

½ cup shredded red cabbage

½ cup shredded green cabbage

1 head endive, trimmed and chopped into bite-size pieces

½ head radicchio, chopped into bite-size pieces

½ cup fresh Italian parsley leaves

½ cup fresh cilantro

½ cup dandelion greens

2 tablespoons olive oil

1 tablespoon lemon-flavored Nordic Naturals Omega-3 Oil

1 teaspoon Dijon mustard

1 teaspoon apple cider vinegar

1 can sardines, for serving (optional)

1. In a large salad bowl, combine the arugula, red and green cabbage, endive, radicchio, parsley, cilantro, and dandelion greens.

2. In a small mixing bowl, combine the olive oil, omega-3 oil, mustard, and vinegar and whisk together until well mixed.

3. Pour the dressing over the greens in the salad bowl and toss with salad tongs. Serve with sardines, if desired.

SWAP: *If you can't find the Nordic Naturals oil, you can simply squeeze the juice of ½ lemon into the dressing and add a teaspoon of MCT oil or other neutral-flavored oil.*

SUPER QUICK

2

SERVINGS

Per Serving: Calories: 288; Total Fat: 28g; Total Carbohydrates: 7g; Net Carbs: 4g; Fiber: 3g; Protein: 2g

Macronutrients: Fat 88%; Protein 2%; Carbs 10%

TRIVIA: *Make this salad if you have digestive issues! Eating bitter foods activates taste buds that stimulate enzyme production and bile flow, which promotes digestion. The high fiber content of this salad also helps with bowel elimination.*

MINESTRONE SOUP

PREP TIME: 20 MINUTES / COOK TIME: 1 HOUR

This soup is basically the keto version of the classic "everything but the kitchen sink"—a recipe to make the most of leftovers. If you've had vegetables sitting in your fridge or freezer for a while and want to finally use them, this delicious soup is your go-to.

BULK COOK, ONE POT

3
SERVINGS

Per Serving: Calories: 359; Total Fat: 24g; Total Carbohydrates: 23g; Net Carbs: 14g; Fiber: 9g; Protein: 15g

Macronutrients: Fat 60%; Protein 15%; Carbs 25%

3 tablespoons olive oil

½ onion, diced

1 carrot, peeled and diced

1 celery stalk, diced

1 cup Brussels sprouts, quartered

1 cup green beans, trimmed

¼ cup tomato paste

2 garlic cloves, minced

1 teaspoon dried basil

1 teaspoon dried marjoram

1 teaspoon dried thyme

½ (15-ounce) can crushed tomatoes with their juices

2 dried bay leaves

¼ to ½ teaspoon red pepper flakes (optional)

2 cups vegetable broth

1 cup water or beef broth

Salt

Freshly ground black pepper

1 cup chopped kale

1 bag Miracle Noodle ziti-shaped noodles (optional)

¾ cup soft goat cheese, for topping

1. Heat the olive oil in a large pot over medium heat. Add the onion, carrot, and celery and cook for about 10 minutes.

2. Add the Brussels sprouts, green beans, tomato paste, and garlic to the pot along with the basil, marjoram, and thyme. Cook for about 3 minutes, stirring constantly.

3. Add the crushed tomatoes and their juices, bay leaves, red pepper flakes (if using), vegetable broth, and water or beef broth. Season with salt and pepper. Stir everything together, reduce the heat to low, and simmer for about 20 minutes.

4. Add the kale to the pot and simmer for another 20 minutes. If using the noodles, add them in the last 2 minutes of cooking. Top with the goat cheese.

5. Let the soup cool for a few minutes before serving or else you will 100 percent burn your mouth!

TIP: *This soup does cook for a long time, but that time is important to let the flavors really shine through.*

SWAP: *If you prefer another green instead of kale, feel free to use it. You can also add extra protein or fat to this recipe, such as chicken or more oil if you need to up your fat quota for the day.*

COBB SALAD

PREP TIME: 15 MINUTES / COOK TIME: 15 MINUTES

The Cobb salad is a classic. While a Cobb salad from a restaurant can contain anywhere from 940 to 1,110 calories, this one is way healthier. The keto diet is not about counting calories, but making this salad at home will help you save some calories to leave room for other tasty recipes from this book!

SUPER QUICK

4
SERVINGS

Per Serving: Calories: 804; Total Fat: 64g; Total Carbohydrates: 13g; Net Carbs: 5g; Fiber: 8g; Protein: 44g

Macronutrients: Fat 72%; Protein 22%; Carbs 6%

1 cup chopped butter lettuce

1 cup chopped romaine lettuce

½ cup chopped iceberg lettuce

2 tomatoes, quartered, or 1 pint cherry tomatoes, halved

2 avocados, halved, pitted, peeled, and diced

2 hard-boiled eggs, quartered

½ cup chopped jicama

1 tablespoon olive oil

1 pound turkey breast or ground turkey

Salt

Freshly ground black pepper

4 slices sugar-free bacon (pork, turkey, beef, or salmon)

½ cup algae oil, or ¼ cup olive oil and ¼ cup MCT oil

1 tablespoon red wine vinegar

1 tablespoon Dijon mustard

Chia seeds, for serving (optional)

Grated cheese of choice, for serving (optional)

1. In a large salad bowl, toss all of the lettuce with the tomatoes, avocados, eggs, and jicama. Set aside.

2. Heat the olive oil in a large skillet over medium-high heat, add the turkey, and cook for 8 to 10 minutes per side. Season with salt and pepper. Transfer the turkey to a plate to cool.

3. In the same skillet, cook the bacon to your desired doneness, about 5 minutes.

4. Chop the turkey and bacon into pieces and add to the salad bowl.

5. In a mixing bowl, stir together the oil, vinegar, and mustard and season with salt and pepper. Pour over the salad and toss with tongs.

6. Divide the Cobb salad evenly among four plates, making sure each person gets about 4 ounces of turkey, 1 slice of bacon, half of a hard-boiled egg, and half of an avocado. If desired, serve sprinkled with chia seeds and/or grated cheese.

TIP: *You can find a lot of these ingredients prechopped at your local grocery store. Feel free to pick up pre-cooked and chopped turkey, tomatoes, eggs, avocados, jicama, and lettuces, as well.*

SWAP: *If you want a nuttier dressing, you can use flaxseed oil.*

ASIAN CUCUMBER SALAD

PREP TIME: 10 MINUTES

I am 100 percent obsessed with Asian food. Sashimi. Hand rolls without the rice. Poke bowls. When I am not writing, you will most likely find my face in a plate full of these foods. A lot of them come paired with a tasty-looking cucumber salad, which I find always looks refreshing yet typically contains sugar. I've replicated the vitamin K–rich salad here for you.

SUPER QUICK

4
SERVINGS

Per Serving: Calories: 148; Total Fat: 12g; Total Carbohydrates: 8g; Net Carbs: 6g; Fiber: 2g; Protein: 2g; Erythritol: 1g

Macronutrients: Fat 73%; Protein 5%; Carbs 22%

TIP: *If you don't feel like chopping up cucumbers and onions for this recipe, you may be able to find them already chopped up in the salad bar at your grocery store.*

SWAP: *If you can't find or don't like seaweed, omit it from the recipe or replace it with spinach or mixed greens.*

2 large cucumbers, sliced into rounds

3 tablespoons seaweed mix (like SeaSnax SeaVegi Seaweed Salad Mix)

½ red onion, diced

½ teaspoon minced garlic or garlic powder

1 teaspoon minced pickled ginger

1 tablespoon tamari or coconut aminos

1 teaspoon erythritol or monk fruit extract

3 tablespoons sesame oil

1 tablespoon sesame seeds

½ teaspoon red pepper flakes (optional)

1 sheet toasted nori (optional)

Salt

Seared ahi tuna or salmon sashimi, for serving

1. In a mixing bowl, combine the cucumbers, seaweed, onion, garlic, ginger, tamari, erythritol, sesame oil, sesame seeds, and red pepper flakes (if using). Season with salt. Mix everything together to evenly coat the cucumbers and seaweed mix.

2. Crumble the toasted nori (if using) over the top of the salad and serve with seared ahi tuna or salmon sashimi.

CAULIFLOWER "POTATO" SALAD

PREP TIME: 10 MINUTES / COOK TIME: 15 MINUTES

Going to a group gathering like a barbecue can be daunting when you're first starting on keto. Is it the people who are daunting? No, no. It's that luscious potato salad that you know you shouldn't eat. Well, I'm so happy to have a solution for you—this mock "potato" salad will be your protection against temptation.

2 cups cauliflower florets

1 tablespoon chopped celery

1 hard-boiled egg, chopped

1½ tablespoons mayonnaise

1 tablespoon sugar-free pickle relish

1 tablespoon mustard

Salt

Freshly ground black pepper

Chopped fresh chives, for garnish

1. Put the cauliflower in a pot, cover with ¼ inch of water, and steam over medium heat for about 10 minutes, or until fork-tender.

2. Let the cauliflower cool, then chop into chunky pieces and put in a mixing bowl.

3. Add the celery, egg, mayonnaise, relish, and mustard, season with salt and pepper, and stir until evenly combined.

4. Sprinkle the salad with chives and serve.

TIP: *Using frozen cauliflower works just fine for this recipe, as well, and you can even just heat it up in the microwave!*

BULK COOK, SUPER QUICK

1-2
SERVINGS

Per Serving: Calories: 319; Total Fat: 23g; Total Carbohydrates: 15g; Net Carbs: 8g; Fiber: 7g; Protein: 12g

Macronutrients: Fat 65%; Protein 15%; Carbs 20%

TRIVIA: *Feel free to add diced red bell peppers to this recipe for a little extra vitamin C!*

LOBSTER BLT SALAD

PREP TIME: 15 MINUTES / COOK TIME: 10 TO 15 MINUTES

You may have heard that lobsters mate for life. Well, unfortunately, that's not actually true. What is true is that you will most likely want to mate for life with this salad rich in selenium (a trace mineral that aids in boosting your immune system) thanks to the sweetness of the lobster meat paired with the crisp saltiness of the bacon and the creamy avocado.

SUPER QUICK

4
SERVINGS

Per Serving: Calories: 436; Total Fat: 28g; Total Carbohydrates: 11g; Net Carbs: 7g; Fiber: 4g; Protein: 35g

Macronutrients: Fat 58%; Protein 32%; Carbs 10%

2 (2½-pound) lobsters
8 slices sugar-free bacon (pork, turkey, beef, or salmon)
2 tablespoons Primal Kitchen mayonnaise (spicy or regular)
1 tablespoon Dijon mustard
1 tablespoon chopped fresh chives
Salt
1 pound butter lettuce, chopped
1 large beefsteak tomato, sliced
1 avocado, halved, pitted, peeled, and sliced

1. Bring a pot of water to a boil.
2. Put the lobsters in the pot, cover, and steam for 5 to 7 minutes per pound.
3. Remove the lobsters from the pot and let cool.
4. While lobsters cool, cook the bacon to your desired doneness, about 5 minutes.
5. When lobster is cool enough to handle, use a sharp knife and a claw cracker to get the meat out. Claw and tail meat are best to use for this recipe. (Save any remaining lobster meat to make seafood stock or to eat as a snack.) Chop the meat into pieces and put in a mixing bowl.

6. Add the mayonnaise, mustard, and chives, season with salt, and mix together.

7. Arrange the butter lettuce, tomato, and avocado on plates. Scoop the lobster mixture alongside and serve with the bacon slices either whole or crumbled and sprinkled on top.

TIP: *Walmart and Costco sell lobster tails in their freezer section. Bar Harbor is also a canned fish company that sells lobster in a can.*

SWAP: *If lobster is not readily available for you, you can always use langoustines, crawfish, or shrimp.*

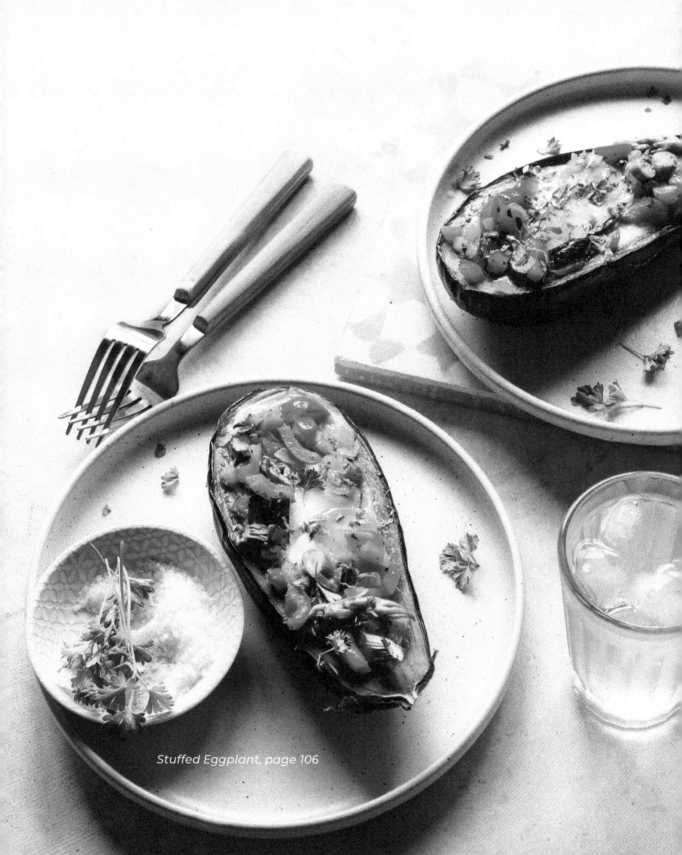

Stuffed Eggplant, page 106

Chapter 6

Vegetarian Main Dishes

Following keto as a vegetarian isn't as challenging as some might think. For those who eat eggs and dairy, it is surprisingly easy, as these recipes demonstrate.

Asparagus & Fennel Frittata 100

Shakshuka 102

Roasted Cabbage "Steaks" 103

Mediterranean Spaghetti 104

Stuffed Eggplant 106

Roasted Brussels Sprouts & Poached Eggs 108

Hearts of Palm Linguine with Butternut Squash
"Cheese" Sauce 110

Fettuccine Alfredo (2 Variations) 111

Cauliflower Mac & Cheese 113

Green Vegetable Stir-Fry with Tofu 114

ASPARAGUS & FENNEL FRITTATA

PREP TIME: 5 TO 10 MINUTES / COOK TIME: 30 MINUTES

The first time I ever had a frittata was at a brunch birthday party for superstar and feminist icon Barbra Streisand. Perhaps she invited me because she wanted to find out what my blog title, GiGi Eats Celebrities, really meant? (It's good to face your fears!) Now, as excited as I was to see Barbra in person, I must admit that I was equally fixated on the frittata that was served. I think if I hadn't been on my best behavior for Barbra, I would have taken the entire egg pie with me to the bathroom and devoured it. I held myself back, though, and took note of the ingredients and flavors so I could craft a frittata of my own just as good that I can eat as much of as I want in the privacy of my own home.

BULK COOK

4
SERVINGS

Per Serving: Calories: 188;
Total Fat: 12g; Total
Carbohydrates: 6g; Net Carbs:
4g; Fiber: 2g; Protein: 14g

Macronutrients: Fat 57%;
Protein 30%; Carbs 13%

1 teaspoon coconut or regular butter, plus more for greasing

8 asparagus spears, diced

½ cup diced fennel

½ cup mushrooms, sliced (optional)

8 eggs

½ cup full-fat regular milk or coconut milk

1 tomato, sliced

1 teaspoon salt

½ teaspoon freshly ground black pepper

Grated cheese (optional)

1. Preheat the oven to 350°F. Grease a pie dish with butter.

2. Melt 1 teaspoon of butter in a shallow skillet over medium-high heat and sauté the asparagus, fennel, and mushrooms (if using) for about 5 minutes, or until fork-tender.

3. Transfer the vegetables to the prepared pie dish.

4. Crack the eggs into a mixing bowl and pour in the milk. Whisk together until fully combined.

5. Pour the egg mixture over the vegetables in the pie dish, season with salt and pepper, and carefully and lightly mix everything together. Lay the tomato slices on top.

6. Bake the frittata for about 30 minutes.

7. Remove from the oven and let cool for 5 to 10 minutes. Slice into wedges and sprinkle with grated cheese, if desired.

SWAP: *If you are not a fan of fennel, you can swap in ½ cup of diced onions.*

SHAKSHUKA

PREP TIME: 30 MINUTES / COOK TIME: 30 TO 40 MINUTES

This recipe will shake your taste buds in an amazing way because it's bursting with spicy North African flavors! On top of that, the combination of herbs and spices is bursting with compounds that aid in digestion, blood sugar control, lowering bad cholesterol levels, and the prevention of foodborne illnesses! This recipe clearly covers all the bases!

BULK COOK, ONE POT

4

SERVINGS

Per Serving: Calories: 232; Total Fat: 16g; Total Carbohydrates: 9g; Net Carbs: 7g; Fiber: 2g; Protein: 13g

Macronutrients: Fat 62%; Protein 22%; Carbs 16%

TIP: *If you prefer a sweeter dish, add more of the "brown sugar" and omit or reduce the red pepper flakes.*

2 tablespoons olive oil

1 small white onion, diced

2 garlic cloves, finely chopped

1 bell pepper, diced (any color)

1½ (15-ounce) cans diced tomatoes

2 tablespoons tomato paste

1 tablespoon paprika

1 teaspoon ground cumin

1 teaspoon red pepper flakes

1 teaspoon salt

½ teaspoon freshly ground black pepper

1 teaspoon erythritol brown "sugar" (optional)

8 eggs

½ bunch fresh cilantro, minced, for garnish

Sugar-free hot sauce, for serving (optional)

Crumbled feta or grated mozzarella or Parmesan cheese, for serving (optional)

1. In a deep sauté pan with a lid, heat the olive oil over medium-high heat. Add the onion and garlic and cook for 3 to 4 minutes. Add the bell pepper, stir, and cook for another 5 minutes.

2. Stir in the canned tomatoes and tomato paste. Add the paprika, cumin, red pepper flakes, salt, pepper, and sweetener (if using) and stir to incorporate.

3. Carefully crack each egg into the pan, making sure not to crack one on top of another.

4. Cover the pan, reduce the heat to medium, and cook for about 20 minutes, or until the eggs are cooked to your desired doneness.

5. Remove from the heat, sprinkle with cilantro, hot sauce, and cheese (if using), and serve warm.

ROASTED CABBAGE "STEAKS"

PREP TIME: 5 MINUTES / COOK TIME: 30 TO 40 MINUTES

Vegetarians can eat steak, too. Okay, not quite, but you will see that the cabbage in this recipe has a nice silky texture and bold flavor thanks to the cooking process, which makes it taste sweeter. It also melts in your mouth, much like a rare piece of steak might.

1 head white or green cabbage, sliced 1 inch thick

4 tablespoons olive oil

1 teaspoon garlic powder

1 teaspoon onion powder

Salt

Freshly ground black pepper

4 eggs, over-easy, for serving (optional)

1. Preheat the oven to 450°F.

2. Put the cabbage pieces on a baking sheet and brush all over with the olive oil. Sprinkle all over with the garlic and onion powder and season with salt and pepper.

3. Roast for 30 to 40 minutes, flipping the cabbage halfway through cooking (you may have to or want to do this several times so the cabbage doesn't burn).

TIP: *Stay near the kitchen while the cabbage is roasting, as it has the potential to burn if it's unattended for too long.*

SWAP: *Purple cabbage can also work for this recipe, but might take 5 to 10 minutes longer to roast than white or green cabbage.*

ONE POT

4
SERVINGS

Per Serving: Calories: 194; Total Fat: 14g; Total Carbohydrates: 14g; Net Carbs: 8g; Fiber: 6g; Protein: 3g

Macronutrients: Fat 65%; Protein 6%; Carbs 29%

MEDITERRANEAN SPAGHETTI

PREP TIME: 10 MINUTES / COOK TIME: 20 MINUTES

In my personal opinion, Mediterranean flavors never bore the palate, which is a great thing because you can make enough of this tasty dish to last you a week or longer! It also makes for a wonderful side dish (if you're finally running low on its leftovers)!

ONE POT, SUPER QUICK

2
SERVINGS

Per Serving: Calories: 430; Total Fat: 26g; Total Carbohydrates: 40g; Net Carbs: 28g; Fiber: 12g; Protein: 9g

Macronutrients: Fat 55%; Protein 9%; Carbs 36%

3 tablespoons olive oil

1 onion, diced

2 garlic cloves, minced

1 cup diced eggplant

2 whole artichoke hearts, quartered

½ (15-ounce) can tomato purée

½ cup olives, pitted and coarsely chopped

2 tablespoons chopped fresh basil leaves

1 tablespoon dried oregano

3 tablespoons capers

1 teaspoon salt

½ teaspoon freshly ground black pepper

½ can tomato paste (optional)

16 ounces cooked spaghetti squash or hearts of palm noodles

Chopped fresh parsley, for serving (optional)

Grated cheese, for serving (optional)

1. In a shallow skillet, heat the olive oil over medium-high heat. Add the onion and garlic and cook for 3 to 5 minutes, stirring, then add the eggplant. Reduce the heat to medium, cook for 5 minutes more, and add the artichoke hearts.

2. Stir everything together, then pour in the tomato purée and add the olives, basil, oregano, capers, salt, and pepper. Cook for another 5 to 8 minutes, adding the tomato paste if you'd like the sauce to be thicker.

3. At this point, you can either add the cooked spaghetti squash directly to the skillet and toss to coat with the sauce, or you can put it on a serving dish and pour the sauce over the top. Sprinkle with parsley and cheese if you'd like, then serve and enjoy!

TIP: *Feel free to make your own tomato sauce, or you can use Rao's Homemade tomato sauces—I recommend the tomato basil, roasted eggplant, or roasted garlic varieties. You can simply warm these sauces up and pour over your spaghetti of choice. Mix in the vegetables in the ingredients list if you need more carbohydrates for the day.*

SWAP: *Shirataki noodles, zucchini noodles, or summer squash noodles can be used in place of the veggie noodles called for.*

STUFFED EGGPLANT

PREP TIME: 20 MINUTES / COOK TIME: 1 HOUR

You may be convinced more than ever to stuff yourself full of eggplant when you learn that it's full of potassium, vitamin C, and B6, which are all wonderful aids for heart health. Eggplant is also magic when it comes to reducing the risk of stroke and heart attack thanks to a flavonoid that has been shown to help reduce blood pressure. Eggplant contains iron and copper, as well, which can boost your energy levels. Clearly this is a dish you can feel good about stuffing yourself with!

2-4
SERVINGS

Per Serving: Calories: 380;
Total Fat: 26g; Total
Carbohydrates: 25g; Net
Carbs: 15g; Fiber: 10g;
Protein: 12g

Macronutrients: Fat 62%;
Protein 12%; Carbs 26%

1 small eggplant, halved lengthwise

3 tablespoons olive, avocado, or macadamia nut oil

1 onion, diced

12 asparagus spears or green beans, diced

1 red bell pepper, diced

1 large tomato, chopped

2 garlic cloves, minced

½ block (8 ounces) extra-firm tofu (optional)

3 tablespoons chopped fresh basil leaves

Salt

Freshly ground black pepper

¼ cup water

2 eggs

Chopped fresh parsley, for garnish (optional)

Shredded cheese, for garnish (optional)

1. Preheat the oven to 350°F.

2. Scoop out the flesh from the halved eggplant and chop it into cubes. Reserve the eggplant skin.

3. In a sauté pan with a lid, heat the oil over medium-high heat. Add the eggplant, onion, asparagus, bell pepper, tomato, garlic, and tofu (if using) and stir. Stir in the basil, season with salt and pepper, and cook for about 5 minutes.

4. Add the water, cover the pan, reduce the heat to medium, and cook for about 15 minutes longer.

5. Put the eggplant "boats" (the reserved skin) on a baking sheet. Scoop some of the cooked eggplant mixture into each boat (you may have some filling left over, which is fine—you can roast it alongside the eggplant).

6. Crack an egg into each eggplant boat, on top of the filling, then bake for about 40 minutes, or until desired doneness.

7. Remove the eggplant from the oven and, if desired, sprinkle parsley and cheese over the top. Let the cheese melt and cool for about 5 minutes, then serve them up!

TIP: *You can throw any vegetable you have on hand into this recipe: leeks, cauliflower, broccoli, cabbage . . . the list goes on. This recipe helps you get rid of veggies that may spoil in the next day or two!*

SWAP: *If you don't like tofu or would prefer to use another vegetarian/vegan meat substitute, feel free to do so, but read ingredients to make sure they're not made with omega-6 oils or wheat products.*

ROASTED BRUSSELS SPROUTS & POACHED EGGS

PREP TIME: 8 MINUTES / COOK TIME: 35 MINUTES

I don't like going to fancy-schmancy restaurants, but there's one that I went to that ended up inspiring this dish. The restaurant had a bunch of side dishes you could choose from and I wound up making my meal out of a few of them—a good tip for all of you, by the way. To this day it may very well be one of my favorite meals I have ever eaten. And, this recipe is just as delicious.

2
SERVINGS

Per Serving: Calories: 310;
Total Fat: 26g; Total
Carbohydrates: 10g; Net
Carbs: 6g; Fiber: 4g;
Protein: 9g

Macronutrients: Fat 75%;
Protein 12%; Carbs 13%

2 cups Brussels sprouts, halved

3 tablespoons olive or avocado oil

1 teaspoon garlic powder

1 teaspoon salt

½ teaspoon freshly ground black pepper

2 eggs

Hollandaise sauce from Eggs Benedict on Grilled Portobello Mushroom Caps (page 54; optional)

¼ teaspoon red pepper flakes (optional)

1. Preheat the oven to 400°F.

2. Put the Brussels sprouts in a bowl, add the oil, and season with garlic powder, salt, and pepper. Stir until the sprouts are evenly coated.

3. Spread the sprouts out evenly on a baking sheet and roast for 30 to 35 minutes, tossing halfway through.

4. When the Brussels sprouts have about 10 more minutes to cook, poach the eggs. Bring a saucepan of water to a boil, then reduce the heat to low. Crack the eggs into a small bowl and carefully pour them into the simmering water. Turn off the heat, cover the pan, and let the eggs cook for about 5 minutes.

5. Remove the Brussels sprouts from the oven and distribute onto plates, about 1 cup per person.

6. Using a slotted spoon, carefully remove the eggs from the water and place on top of the sprouts.

7. Drizzle hollandaise sauce over the top if you wish, then sprinkle with the red pepper flakes, which are completely optional but delicious!

TIP: *Some grocery stores (like Trader Joe's) have pre-roasted Brussels sprouts in their produce department if you don't feel like making your own. Warm them up in the oven or air fryer if you have one.*

SWAP: *If you don't want to go through the hassle of poaching eggs, over-easy eggs are just as delicious and still give you that runny yolk that truly defines the dish.*

HEARTS OF PALM LINGUINE WITH BUTTERNUT SQUASH "CHEESE" SAUCE

PREP TIME: 5 MINUTES / COOK TIME: 10 MINUTES

There was a time in my life when I refused to eat anything green. A favorite story that gets retold by my family is from a time we were traveling in France. At a restaurant, I ordered spaghetti with butter and Parmesan cheese. The restaurant tried to liven up my dish by sprinkling a little parsley on top. When it arrived, mayhem ensued. Thankfully my palate and my manners have matured since then! Now I adore this play on traditional spaghetti, sprinkled with lots of parsley. Oh, and don't worry, I have apologized to my family profusely for my parsley-related tantrum.

ONE POT, SUPER QUICK

2
SERVINGS

Per Serving: Calories: 342;
Total Fat: 18g; Total
Carbohydrates: 22g; Net
Carbs: 15g; Fiber: 7g;
Protein: 23g

Macronutrients: Fat 50%;
Protein 25%; Carbs 25%

TRIVIA: *One cup of parsley provides about 1,230 percent of the recommended daily allowance of vitamin K!*

½ recipe Butternut Squash "Cheese" Sauce (page 216)

1 cup of shredded Cheddar cheese

2 (14-ounce) cans hearts of palm linguine, rinsed and drained

Salt

Freshly ground black pepper

Chopped fresh parsley, for serving (optional but highly recommended)

1. In a large pot, warm the Butternut Squash "Cheese" Sauce and Cheddar over medium heat for 5 minutes. Add the hearts of palm linguine and stir to incorporate. Cook for 5 minutes more to warm through.

2. Serve the pasta in bowls, season with salt and pepper, and sprinkle with fresh parsley, if desired.

SWAP: *If you don't like hearts of palm, use shirataki noodles (such as Miracle Noodle brand), or noodles made from zucchini, summer squash, or butternut squash.*

BRAND: *Palmini Pasta is a brand of hearts of palm pasta, as is Natural Heaven. You can also buy regular cans of hearts of palm and slice them up into noodles yourself—easy-peasy.*

FETTUCCINE ALFREDO (2 VARIATIONS)

PREP TIME: 5 MINUTES / COOK TIME: 10 MINUTES

My husband's diet sometimes looks like that of a nine-year-old. I say this with love, but it's true. He eats whatever he wants, whenever he wants. One of his favorite foods is fettuccine Alfredo with chicken and broccoli. While I commend him for the chicken and broccoli, the rest can't be stomached by yours truly or anyone else following a keto lifestyle. That is, until now.

FOR BOTH VARIATIONS

2 (7-ounce) packages shirataki noodles or 5 cups spaghetti squash or hearts of palm noodles

1 tablespoon chopped fresh parsley, chives, or basil, for serving (optional)

FOR THE DAIRY VARIATION

2 tablespoons grass-fed/-finished butter or ghee

2 teaspoons garlic powder or 2 small garlic cloves, minced

1½ cups grass-fed/-finished heavy (whipping) cream

1 cup grated Parmesan cheese

Salt

Freshly ground black pepper

FOR THE VEGAN VARIATION

2 tablespoons butter-flavored coconut oil

2 teaspoons garlic powder or 2 small garlic cloves, minced

1½ cups heavy coconut cream (shake the can well before measuring)

4 tablespoons nutritional yeast

Salt

Freshly ground black pepper

ONE POT, SUPER QUICK

4–6
SERVINGS

Per Serving: Calories: 510; Total Fat: 46g; Total Carbohydrates: 12g; Net Carbs: 10g; Fiber: 2g; Protein: 12g

Macronutrients: Fat 81%; Protein 10%; Carbs 9%

1. If you're making the dairy version, melt the butter in a skillet over medium heat, add the garlic, and stir together. Add the cream and cheese, season with salt and pepper, and whisk everything together. Cook for about 10 minutes, or until the cheese is melted.

2. If you're making the vegan version, melt the coconut oil in a skillet over medium heat, add the garlic, and stir together. Add the coconut cream and nutritional yeast, season with salt and pepper, and whisk everything together. Cook for about 10 minutes.

FETTUCCINE ALFREDO (2 VARIATIONS) *continues*

BRAND: *Vital Farms is my favorite brand for grass-fed butter, and Organic Valley has a great grass-fed heavy (whipping) cream. There are also lots of great brands of shirataki noodles on the market these days in addition to Miracle Noodle—just make sure to read the ingredients labels.*

SWAP: *You can always use noodles made from zucchini, summer squash, or butternut squash, if you prefer.*

3. Add the noodles to the skillet and cook, stirring, for 1 minute to coat in the sauce.

4. Dish up in bowls and sprinkle with chopped parsley, chives, or basil, if desired.

TIP: *If you want the dairy-laden sauce but don't want to make it yourself, you can use Rao's Homemade Alfredo sauce.*

CAULIFLOWER MAC & CHEESE

PREP TIME: 5 MINUTES / COOK TIME: 15 MINUTES

When I was growing up, I loved boxed macaroni and cheese. My mother, however, certainly did not allow it in our house because of how unhealthy it is. Obviously, I found my way around that by eating loads of it at my friends' houses. Nowadays I don't have to sneak around or feel guilty. I can happily wreak havoc on this recipe because I know I'm feeding myself the best of the best.

1 small head cauliflower, coarsely chopped

1 recipe Cheese Sauce (from Nachos, page 76) or Butternut Squash "Cheese" Sauce (for vegan; page 216)

Salt

Freshly ground black pepper

Chopped fresh parsley, for serving (optional)

Sugar-free hot sauce, for serving (optional)

1. In a deep pot with a lid, cover the cauliflower with about ¼ inch of water. Cover the pot, turn the stove to medium heat, and let the cauliflower steam for 5 to 7 minutes.

2. Turn off the heat and let the cauliflower continue to steam.

3. Meanwhile, in a saucepan, warm the cheese sauce over low heat for a few minutes.

4. Using a slotted spoon, remove the cauliflower from the pot and divide between two bowls. Spoon or pour cheese sauce evenly over the cauliflower and stir together.

5. Season with salt and pepper, sprinkle with parsley (if using), and top with hot sauce if you'd like.

BULK COOK, SUPER QUICK

2
SERVINGS

Per Serving: Calories: 343; Total Fat: 15g; Total Carbohydrates: 37g; Net Carbs: 23g; Fiber: 14g; Protein: 15g

Macronutrients: Fat 40%; Protein 18%; Carbs 42%

TRIVIA: *While a lot of people assume vegetables have more nutrition the deeper in color they are, cauliflower is jam-packed with essential vitamins and minerals. Vitamin K, which supports your bones, and vitamin C, which aids in immune health and collagen production, are two shining stars in this vegetable.*

GREEN VEGETABLE STIR-FRY WITH TOFU

PREP TIME: 15 MINUTES / COOK TIME: 15 MINUTES

If you suffer from allergies, this salad could very well be a wonderful substitute for your sea-sonal allergy medication, because it's loaded with quercetin (thanks to the onion and leek), a natural antihistamine! Eat this stir-fry enough, and maybe you won't have to worry about what the changing seasons do to your sinuses!

**ONE POT,
SUPER QUICK**

2

SERVINGS

Per Serving: Calories: 473;
Total Fat: 33g; Total
Carbohydrates: 27g; Net
Carbs: 15g; Fiber: 12g;
Protein: 17g

Macronutrients: Fat 63%;
Protein 15%; Carbs 22%

3 tablespoons avocado oil, divided

1 cup Brussels sprouts, halved

½ onion, diced

½ leek, white and light green parts diced

½ head green cabbage, diced

¼ cup water, plus more if needed

½ cup kale, coarsely chopped

1 cup spinach, coarsely chopped

8 ounces tofu, diced

2 teaspoons garlic powder

Salt

Freshly ground black pepper

½ avocado, pitted, peeled, and diced

MCT oil (optional)

1. In a large skillet with a lid (or a wok if you have one), heat 2 tablespoons of avocado oil over medium-high heat. Add the Brussels sprouts, onion, leek, and cabbage and stir together. Add the water, cover, lower the heat to medium, and cook for about 5 minutes.

2. Toss in the kale and spinach and cook for 3 minutes, stirring constantly, until the onion, leek, and cabbage are caramelized.

3. Add the tofu to the stir-fry, then season with the garlic, salt, pepper, and the remaining tablespoon of avocado oil.

4. Turn the heat back up to medium-high and cook for about 10 minutes, stirring constantly, until the tofu is nice and caramelized on all sides. If you experience any burning, turn down the heat and add 2 to 3 tablespoons of water.

5. Divide the stir-fry between two plates and sprinkle with diced avocado. Feel free to drizzle algae oil or MCT oil over the top for a little extra fat.

SWAP: *You can use 3 or 4 eggs in this recipe instead of tofu if you'd prefer to steer clear of soy.*

TRIVIA: *Always make sure you purchase organic soy products, because soy is often genetically modified. While more studies are necessary, genetically modified processed soy has been linked to issues affecting women, including infertility and immune system and insulin-regulating problems.*

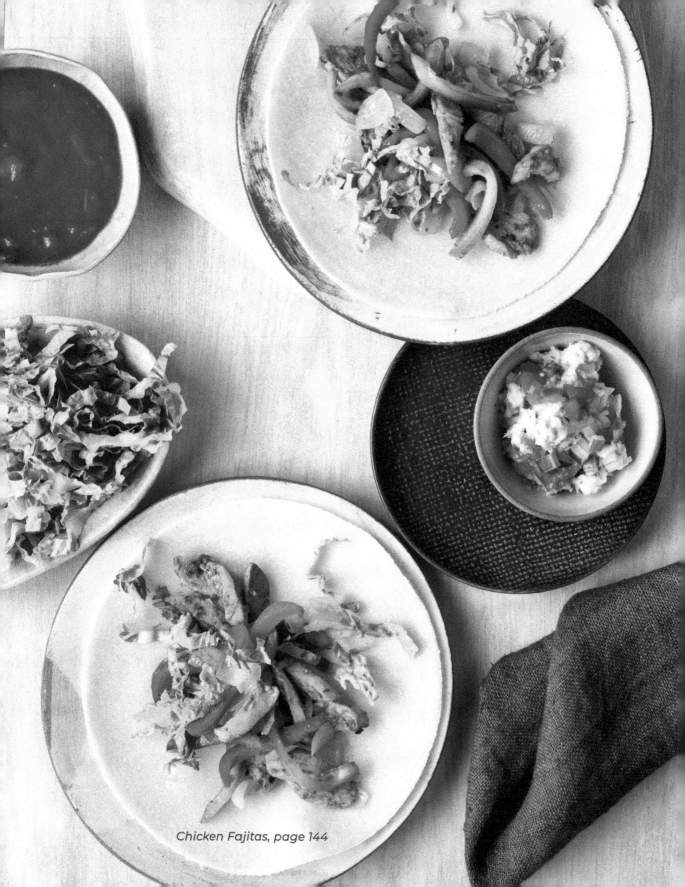

Chicken Fajitas, page 144

Chapter 7

Seafood & Poultry

In my opinion, the following recipes are clucking delicious and will hopefully have you swimming back for more, because B vitamins, potassium, selenium, zinc, and omega-3 fatty acids, which all of these recipes contain, are essential for your health!

Salmon Poke **118**

Sesame-Crusted Tuna **119**

Salmon with Mustard Sauce **120**

Spaghetti Squash Puttanesca **122**

Mayo-Less Tuna Salad **124**

Simply Broiled or Air-Fried Salmon **125**

Whole Roasted Sea Bass **126**

Sushi **127**

Halibut Curry **129**

Chicken Teriyaki **131**

Chicken Shawarma **133**

Almond Meal–Crusted Chicken Fingers **135**

Meatloaf Muffins **137**

Mezze Cake **139**

Avocado "Toast" **141**

Turkey-Stuffed Avocados **143**

Chicken Fajitas **144**

SALMON POKE

PREP TIME: 5 MINUTES

Whenever my husband asks me what I want for lunch or dinner, hunks of raw salmon dance the Macarena in my brain. All day I dream about my beloved omega-3 fatty acids. My husband and I tend to indulge in my constant craving by heading to our closest poke shop, but now that I've created and mastered this Salmon Poke recipe, I'd rather make it at home.

**ONE POT,
SUPER QUICK**

2

SERVINGS

Per Serving: Calories: 177;
Total Fat: 9g; Total
Carbohydrates: 1g; Net Carbs:
1g; Fiber: 0g; Protein: 23g

Macronutrients: Fat 50%;
Protein 52%; Carbs 8%

½ pound sushi-grade salmon, chopped into ½-inch cubes

¼ small red onion, finely chopped

1 tablespoon dried chives

½ tablespoon capers

1 tablespoon dried basil

1 teaspoon Dijon mustard

½ teaspoon olive oil

Juice of ½ small lemon

Salt

Freshly ground black pepper

1 cucumber, sliced into rounds, for serving (optional)

1. Put the salmon, red onion, and chives in a mixing bowl. Add the capers, basil, mustard, olive oil, and lemon juice and season with salt and pepper. Mix the contents of the bowl together until everything is evenly coated.

2. If desired, spoon the poke onto cucumber rounds (enough to cover the cucumber slice, but not so much that it's falling off). You can certainly eat this poke by itself, too, though.

TIP: *Always make sure to ask the fishmonger if the sushi-grade fish you're buying has been prefrozen. Freezing the fish before thawing (to serve raw) kills off any parasites that may be lurking in it.*

SWAP: *You can use a whitefish like cod or halibut for this recipe if you're not a fan of salmon. Scallops would also work.*

SESAME-CRUSTED TUNA

PREP TIME: 5 MINUTES / COOK TIME: 10 MINUTES

You may only think of sesame seeds as a topping for bagels, but they are far more than that. Sesame seeds are high in vitamins E and K and magnesium. All three of these necessary nutrients contribute to the prevention of inflammation in our bodies and lower the risk of cancer. It's time to incorporate these seeds into your diet far more, don't you think? Let's start now!

¼ cup black and white sesame seeds

Salt

Freshly ground black pepper

1 pound sushi-grade ahi tuna, cut into 2 or 3 equal pieces

2 tablespoons avocado oil

Asian Cucumber Salad (page 94), for serving

1. Pour the sesame seeds into a shallow dish, season with salt and pepper, and mix together to incorporate.

2. Dredge the tuna in the sesame seeds, turning to evenly coat all sides.

3. Heat the oil in a nonstick skillet over medium-high heat.

4. Lay the tuna in the pan and let cook for 3 to 5 minutes, depending on how thick your fillet is and your desired doneness. Flip the tuna over and cook for another 3 to 5 minutes.

5. Serve the tuna with the cucumber salad.

TIP: *Be careful during the cooking process, as sesame seeds tend to pop while cooking and can burn you. It's a good idea to make sure the heat of your stove doesn't go above medium-high.*

SWAP: *If you're not a fan of tuna, you can use salmon, snapper, or mahi-mahi.*

SUPER QUICK

2-3
SERVINGS

Per Serving: Calories: 340; Total Fat: 24g; Total Carbohydrates: 4g; Net Carbs: 2g; Fiber: 2g; Protein: 30g

Macronutrients: Fat 64%; Protein 35%; Carbs 1%

SALMON WITH MUSTARD SAUCE

PREP TIME: 10 MINUTES / COOK TIME: 25 TO 40 MINUTES

Mustard is a girl's best friend in the keto condiment world. Not only is it sugar-free and low in carbohydrates and calories, but it has also been shown to protect against the toxic effect of carcinogens. Oh, and what do you know, salmon is also high in sleep-promoting magnesium, so basically this recipe is a girl's best sleep aid, too.

2-4
SERVINGS

Per Serving: Calories: 333;
Total Fat: 25g; Total
Carbohydrates: 2g; Net Carbs:
2g; Fiber: 0g; Protein: 25g

Macronutrients: Fat 68%;
Protein 30%; Carbs 2%

3 tablespoons olive oil, divided

2 tablespoons Dijon mustard

1 teaspoon freshly squeezed lemon juice

1 shallot, chopped

1 teaspoon minced garlic

¼ cup white wine, such as pinot grigio

Salt

Freshly ground black pepper

1 pound skin-on salmon fillet, cut into 2 to 4 equal pieces

1 teaspoon dried dill

Steamed or grilled leeks or asparagus, or Roasted Cabbage "Steaks" (page 103), for serving

1. Preheat the oven to 400°F. Grease a baking dish with 1 tablespoon of oil.

2. In a food processor, combine the remaining 2 tablespoons of olive oil with the mustard, lemon juice, shallot, garlic, and white wine, season with salt and pepper, and process until smooth.

3. Lay the salmon on the prepared baking dish, then pour the mustard sauce over the top, making sure the entire fillet is covered (you can use a spoon for this if you'd prefer). Sprinkle with the dill.

4. Bake the salmon for 25 to 40 minutes, depending on the type of salmon you use and your desired doneness (see Tip).

5. Serve the salmon with a side of steamed or grilled veggies or the cabbage "steaks."

TIP: *The reason the timing varies in terms of cooking this recipe is that it depends on the type of salmon you purchase. Wild-caught salmon is far less fatty than farmed salmon and will cook in under 25 minutes. Also, if you prefer your salmon a little undercooked, you would only need to cook it for about 25 minutes, as well.*

SWAP: *You can easily swap chicken in for the salmon in this recipe. The fat content will be substantially less, though, even if you go with chicken thighs or legs, so be sure to add more fat to the rest of your day.*

SPAGHETTI SQUASH PUTTANESCA

PREP TIME: 10 MINUTES / COOK TIME: 1 HOUR

When I travel home to visit my parents, my dad has a mini Rolodex of the recipes that he and I make together. Puttanesca sauce is one recipe that I am head over heels in love with, especially when I use it as a spaghetti squash topper. Puttanesca is an Italian sauce invented back in the 1700s that is well-known for its powerfully pungent aroma. I have absolutely no doubt that this combination of olives, tomatoes, capers, garlic, and anchovies all atop a warm bed of spaghetti squash will have you head over heels in love, as well!

2–4
SERVINGS

Per Serving: Calories: 333; Total Fat: 25g; Total Carbohydrates: 17g; Net Carbs: 7g; Fiber: 10g; Protein: 10g

Macronutrients: Fat 68%; Protein 14%; Carbs 18%

1 small spaghetti squash, halved lengthwise and seeded

2 tablespoons olive oil

½ medium yellow onion, finely chopped

Salt

Freshly ground black pepper

1 cup chunky no-sugar-added tomato sauce

½ can halved artichoke hearts, drained

14 olives, pitted and chopped

Splash balsamic vinegar (optional)

1 (2-ounce) can anchovies packed in olive oil

1 (5-ounce) can tuna packed in olive oil

2 tablespoons dried oregano

1 tablespoon capers

1 teaspoon garlic powder

Chopped fresh parsley, for serving (optional)

Grated cheese, for serving (optional)

1. Preheat the oven to 400°F.

2. Place the squash, cut-side down, on a baking sheet and roast in the oven for 45 minutes to 1 hour, or until tender when pierced with a knife.

3. Meanwhile, in a shallow sauté pan or pot, heat the olive oil over medium heat. Add the onion, season with salt and pepper, and cook for about 5 minutes, or until the onion is translucent.

4. Add the tomato sauce and artichoke hearts to the pan and stir together, then stir in the olives and balsamic vinegar (if using).

5. Add the anchovies to the pot, along with the olive oil they're packed in. (There is no need to chop the anchovies because they will disintegrate during the cooking process.)

6. Add the tuna and its oil, the oregano, capers, and garlic powder and stir until everything is completely blended. Cook for another 10 minutes.

7. When the spaghetti squash is done roasting, let cool for 10 to 15 minutes, then scoop puttanesca sauce into each squash half. If you're only serving two people, one half of squash makes the perfect portion size. If you plan on serving four, feel free to cut the squash halves in half again (or scoop the strands out of the squash's shell) and distribute the sauce evenly among each portion.

8. Sprinkle with parsley and cheese, if desired, and serve.

TIP: *Many grocery stores carry precut spaghetti squash in their produce section. All you have to do is microwave it, which will reduce your cooking time tremendously.*

SWAP: *Make this recipe vegetarian by omitting the anchovies and tuna and using tofu instead.*

MAYO-LESS TUNA SALAD

PREP TIME: 5 MINUTES

I personally believe that it's a sin to drain a can of tuna that's packed in olive oil. That olive oil is packed with flavor and loads of health benefits! The monounsaturated fats in it are known to help prevent strokes and heart disease, and even lubricate your joints. Instead of discarding all that goodness, pour all of the can's contents into your mixing bowl for this recipe. If you want to eat with your hands, you can wrap the salad in nori sheets for some iodine-filled crunch!

BULK COOK, SUPER QUICK

1

SERVING

Per Serving: Calories: 450; Total Fat: 38g; Total Carbohydrates: 9g; Net Carbs: 5g; Fiber: 4g; Protein: 18g

Macronutrients: Fat 76%; Protein 16%; Carbs 8%

SWAP: *Canned salmon, sardines, and mackerel work well in place of the tuna.*

1 can tuna packed in olive oil
5 olives, pitted and chopped
4 sun-dried tomatoes, chopped
2 tablespoons chopped jicama
1 tablespoon olive oil
1 teaspoon mustard
1 teaspoon dried basil (optional)
Salt
Freshly ground black pepper
1 cup fresh spinach leaves
Sugar-free hot sauce, for serving (optional)

1. In a mixing bowl, combine the tuna and its oil with the olives, sun-dried tomatoes, jicama, olive oil, and mustard. Season with the basil (if using), salt, and pepper. Stir everything together until well combined.

2. Arrange the spinach leaves on a plate or in a bowl and top with the tuna salad. Or simply toss the spinach with the tuna salad to save yourself a little bit of cleanup! If you'd like, sprinkle with some hot sauce.

TIP: *Always have canned or jarred fish available for quick and easy meals like this one. When you're in a bind, this can save you from turning to something that's not keto-approved.*

SIMPLY BROILED OR AIR-FRIED SALMON

PREP TIME: 5 MINUTES / COOK TIME: 30 MINUTES

I eat salmon one way or another every single day. It never disappoints me, ever, and this fool-proof recipe makes a quick dinner that will totally impress guests, too. It's delicious, but on top of that, salmon is rich in omega-3 fatty acids and high in B vitamins. It also contains an antioxidant that aids in reducing bad cholesterol in your blood.

1 tablespoon olive, avocado, or macadamia nut oil

1 pound salmon fillet or steak (with or without skin), cut into 2 to 4 equal pieces

Salt

Freshly ground black pepper

Dried herbs and spices of your choice (optional)

Steamed or roasted asparagus or spaghetti squash, for serving

ONE POT

2–4
SERVINGS

Per Serving: Calories: 258; Total Fat: 18g; Total Carbohydrates: 0g; Net Carbs: 0g; Fiber: 0g; Protein: 24g

Macronutrients: Fat 63%; Protein 37%; Carbs 0%

1. Preheat the broiler. Line a broiling pan with aluminum foil and grease with the oil. If air-frying, line the air fryer basket with foil and grease with the oil.

2. Season the salmon with salt, pepper, and any other herbs and spices you'd like. Then lay it in the broiling pan (skin-side down, if applicable) or place it in the air-fryer basket.

3. Broil the salmon in the oven for about 30 minutes, checking for doneness (it should form a crisp crust) after about 20 minutes, or cook in the air fryer at 400°F for 25 to 30 minutes. To crisp up skin in the broiler, flip the salmon when there are about 5 minutes left of cooking.

4. Serve the salmon with steamed or roasted vegetables.

SWAP: *You can use this easy cooking method for all types of fish. The fattier the fish, the longer it will take to cook; the leaner the fish, the less time it will take.*

TRIVIA: *If you've ever worried about eating fish due to mercury, fret not. Seafood contains selenium, a mineral that binds with mercury and carries it out of the body. It's still smart to check with your doctor if you have concerns about mercury levels, but the benefits of fish almost always outweigh the negatives.*

WHOLE ROASTED SEA BASS

PREP TIME: 15 MINUTES / COOK TIME: 25 MINUTES

A crispy exterior with a moist and succulent interior—who doesn't love a texture profile like that? This recipe for roasted sea bass covers both of those bases! On top of that, you will be ingesting roughly 16 percent of your daily recommended iron for the day, which aids in energy production, and we could all use a little more energy, no?

ONE POT

4
SERVINGS

Per Serving: Calories: 307; Total Fat: 19g; Total Carbohydrates: 8g; Net Carbs: 5g; Fiber: 3g; Protein: 26g

Macronutrients: Fat 56%; Protein 34%; Carbs 10%

SWAP: *If you're not a lemon fan, you can omit it completely from the recipe. Citrus makes this dish's flavors truly pop, so try using lime instead.*

2 whole sea bass (about 2 pounds), cleaned and scaled

2 tablespoons olive or avocado oil

Salt

Freshly ground black pepper

1 small red onion, sliced into rounds

3 lemons, sliced into rounds

1 large leek, white and light green parts sliced into rounds

8 dried bay leaves

3 tablespoons fresh oregano

Nut-Free Pesto (page 212), for serving (optional)

1. Preheat the oven to 425°F.

2. Put the fish in a shallow baking dish and, using a food brush, brush the fish with the oil. Season with salt and pepper.

3. Fill the cavity of each fish with the onion, lemon, and leek slices, and the bay leaves and oregano.

4. Roast the fish in the oven for about 25 minutes, or until the skin is crispy and the fish is flaky.

5. To serve, remove the head and tail, then cut the fish into 4 equal-size fillets. Serve with Nut-Free Pesto, if desired.

TIP: *When buying whole fish, talk to the fishmonger to make sure it's completely gutted and cleaned, or else you may be left with that task, and it's not an easy one.*

SUSHI

PREP TIME: 15 MINUTES / COOK TIME: 3 TO 5 MINUTES

Making sushi at home is not as hard or daunting as it seems. And I promise it will be far cheaper than going out to a restaurant. I used to go out for sushi a lot—seriously, at least five times a week—and making it at home has saved me a pretty penny. Plus, now I know exactly what's going into everything I eat.

4 cups cauliflower rice

2 tablespoons grass-fed/-finished gelatin

1 tablespoon apple cider vinegar

1 teaspoon salt

2 to 4 nori sheets

½ pound sushi-grade fish, thinly sliced

1 small avocado, halved, pitted, peeled, and thinly sliced

1 small cucumber (or any other vegetable you'd like), thinly sliced

Sesame seeds, for topping (optional)

Coconut aminos or tamari, wasabi, sugar-free pickled ginger, sliced avocado, and/or avocado oil mayonnaise mixed with sugar-free hot sauce, for serving (optional)

SUPER QUICK

2-4
SERVINGS

Per Serving: Calories: 295; Total Fat: 15g; Total Carbohydrates: 10g; Net Carbs: 2g; Fiber: 8g; Protein: 30g

Macronutrients: Fat 46%; Protein 41%; Carbs 13%

1. In a shallow pot with a lid, combine the cauliflower with 3 tablespoons of water. Turn the heat to medium, cover the pot, and steam for 3 to 5 minutes.

2. Drain the cauliflower and transfer to a mixing bowl. Stir in the gelatin, vinegar, and salt. Stir together until the mixture is smooth and sticky. Set aside.

3. Fold a dish towel in half lengthwise and place it on your counter. Cover the towel in plastic wrap.

4. Place a nori sheet on top of the plastic wrap, then spread with a layer of the cauliflower rice.

5. Layer slices of fish, avocado, and cucumber over the cauliflower on the end of the nori sheet closest to you.

SUSHI *continues*

SWAP: *If you're not a fan of nori, you can use coconut wraps, butter lettuce, or cabbage leaves instead.*

TRIVIA: *Both apple cider vinegar and ginger aid in digestion and combat nausea and bloating.*

6. Starting at the end closest to you, gently roll the nori sheet over all the ingredients, using the towel as your rolling aid. (Emphasis on the word "gently" because you don't want to tear the nori sheet.) When you're done rolling, remove the towel and plastic wrap as you slide the roll onto a plate or cutting board. Using a sharp knife, cut the roll into equal pieces. Repeat steps 4 through 7 with the remaining nori and filling ingredients.

7. Sprinkle sesame seeds on top of your sushi, if desired, and serve with any of the other optional ingredients you'd like.

TIP: *You can buy sushi-grade fish from most local Asian supermarkets or high-quality fish markets. Always be sure to ask about the quality and care because sushi-grade fish needs to be frozen prior to use in order to kill any potential parasites.*

HALIBUT CURRY

PREP TIME: 5 MINUTES / COOK TIME: 35 MINUTES

If someone were to ask me what my top five favorite meals of all time are, the curry I ate when I was traveling through Cambodia would certainly rank up there. I had never had curry before my trip, but that first bite catapulted my taste buds into a flavor domain that had me eating a fourth portion, and devouring every bite with a huge smile on my face. When I returned home, I immediately ventured into the kitchen to try and re-create the blissful feast. While mine is not exactly the same, I was able to make something so close to what I had eaten there, I stopped looking up airline tickets back!

1 tablespoon avocado oil

½ cup finely chopped celery

½ cup frozen butternut squash cubes

1 cup full-fat coconut milk

½ cup seafood stock

1½ tablespoons curry powder

1 tablespoon dried cilantro

½ tablespoon garlic powder

½ tablespoon ground turmeric

1 teaspoon ground ginger

1 pound skinless halibut fillet, cut into chunks

Cooked cauliflower rice, for serving (optional)

1. In a large pot with a lid, heat the avocado oil over medium-high heat. Add the celery and cook for about 3 minutes. Add the squash and cook for 5 minutes more.

2. Pour in the coconut milk and seafood stock and cook, stirring, for another 3 minutes. Stir in the curry powder, cilantro, garlic, turmeric, and ginger.

HALIBUT CURRY *continues*

BULK COOK, ONE POT

4
SERVINGS

Per Serving: Calories: 362; Total Fat: 22g; Total Carbohydrates: 8g; Net Carbs: 5g; Fiber: 3g; Protein: 33g

Macronutrients: Fat 55%; Protein 36%; Carbs 9%

SWAP: *Instead of hal-ibut, you can use cod, turbot, haddock, or sole.*

TRIVIA: *Can't find seafood stock at the grocery store? Head to the fish counter and see if they have any fresh or frozen stock in back.*

3. Add the halibut to the pot and stir into the rest of the mixture. Reduce the heat to medium, cover the pot, and cook for 15 to 20 minutes, or until the fish is completely white and flakes easily with a fork.

4. Serve the halibut curry over cauliflower rice if you'd like, or just eat it by itself!

TIP: *Make this recipe in bulk and freeze for future use. It tastes better as leftovers because the flavors will mingle.*

CHICKEN TERIYAKI

PREP TIME: 5 MINUTES (PLUS 1 TO 24 HOURS OF MARINATING TIME) /
COOK TIME: 35 MINUTES

My sister-in-law loves chicken teriyaki but never realized how much sugar it can contain until she met me. I created this sugar-free chicken teriyaki recipe just for her—and now it's for you, as well!

2 pounds boneless, skin-on chicken breasts and thighs

2 tablespoons olive oil

⅓ cup erythritol

¼ cup tamari

1 teaspoon freshly squeezed lemon juice

½ teaspoon garlic powder

¼ teaspoon ground ginger

⅓ cup water

2 tablespoons psyllium husk powder (optional but recommended)

Cooked cauliflower rice, for serving (optional)

Asian Cucumber Salad (page 94), for serving (optional)

BULK COOK

4
SERVINGS

Per Serving: Calories: 452; Total Fat: 32g; Total Carbohydrates: 1g; Net Carbs: 1g; Fiber: 0g; Protein: 40g; Erythritol: 18g

Macronutrients: Fat 64%; Protein 35%; Carbs 1%

1. Put the chicken pieces in a mixing bowl and add the olive oil, erythritol, tamari, lemon juice, garlic, ginger, water, and psyllium husk powder (if using) and mix everything together.

2. Transfer the entire contents of the bowl to a large resealable plastic bag, seal, and shake to make sure the chicken is evenly coated. Let marinate in the refrigerator for at least 1 hour or up to 24 hours. The longer you marinate the chicken, the more flavorful it becomes.

3. When there are 15 to 20 minutes of marinating left, preheat the oven to 400°F and line a baking dish with aluminum foil.

CHICKEN TERIYAKI *continues*

SWAP: *Sick of chicken? You can actually make this entire recipe using turkey breast and thigh, or even ground turkey. Teriyaki turkey burgers, anyone?*

4. Remove the chicken from the marinade (discard the marinade) and place in the prepared baking dish, making sure the pieces don't touch.

5. Roast the chicken for about 30 minutes, flipping halfway through, until cooked all the way through— check by using a sharp knife to make a small incision in the thickest part of one of the pieces.

6. Serve the chicken with cauliflower rice and/or cucumber salad, if desired.

TIP: *If you have an air fryer, you can make this recipe in there using the same heat and time.*

CHICKEN SHAWARMA

PREP TIME: 5 MINUTES (PLUS 2 TO 24 HOURS OF MARINATING TIME) /
COOK TIME: 30 MINUTES

It's rather apparent that this girl loves herself some salmon. Well, consider chicken shawarma to be my salmon of the chicken world. When I am not eating salmon, I am eating chicken sha-warma and making the same loud, happy noises while eating it as I would my beloved pink fish! Shawarma is a Middle Eastern meat preparation that can be made from turkey, chicken, lamb, pork, and beef. The meat is packed together with herbs and spices, roasted on a vertical spit, and then shaved and served with traditional side dishes such as hummus, cucumbers and tomatoes, and rice.

1½ pounds boneless, skinless chicken breast

1 pound skinless chicken thighs

⅓ cup olive oil, divided

2 teaspoons paprika

1 teaspoon allspice

¾ teaspoon ground turmeric

¼ teaspoon garlic powder

¼ teaspoon ground cinnamon

Pinch cayenne pepper

Salt

Freshly ground black pepper

Leafy greens, for serving (optional)

Bean-Free Hummus (page 211), for serving (optional but recommended)

Cooked cauliflower rice, for serving (optional)

BULK COOK

6
SERVINGS

Per Serving: Calories: 410;
Total Fat: 30g; Total
Carbohydrates: 0g; Net Carbs:
0g; Fiber: 0g; Protein: 35g

Macronutrients: Fat 66%;
Protein 34%; Carbs 0%

CHICKEN SHAWARMA *continues*

TIP: *This recipe is great if you're hosting a dinner party and need to feed a lot of people. Or you can make this recipe in bulk and freeze it for future meals. It thaws and reheats deliciously.*

SWAP: *If you are in the mood for red meat, feel free to use steak or lamb for this recipe. Instead of cooking the steak in the oven, go directly from marinating to sautéing in a skillet. You can also use ground meat.*

TRIVIA: *If you ever decide to go out for chicken shawarma, be sure to ask your server or the person at the counter what exactly goes into the recipe, because they sometimes add flour.*

1. Put the chicken breast and thighs in a mixing bowl. Add all but 1 tablespoon of the olive oil, the paprika, allspice, turmeric, garlic powder, cinnamon, cayenne, salt, and pepper and mix everything together.

2. Transfer the entire contents of the bowl to a large resealable plastic bag, seal, and shake to make sure the chicken is evenly coated. Let marinate in the refrigerator for at least 2 hours or up to 24 hours. The longer you marinate the chicken, the more flavorful it becomes.

3. When there are 15 to 20 minutes of marinating left, preheat the oven to 400°F and line a baking dish with aluminum foil.

4. Remove the chicken from the marinade and place in the prepared baking dish, making sure the pieces don't touch.

5. Bake the chicken, flipping at least once, until no longer pink inside, 15 to 20 minutes.

6. Remove the chicken from the oven and, when cool enough to handle, transfer to a cutting board and slice into thin strips.

7. Heat the remaining 1 tablespoon of olive oil in a skillet over medium-high heat and add the chicken strips. Cook for 5 to 7 minutes, or until crispy.

8. If desired, serve the chicken shawarma on a bed of leafy greens, paired with Bean-Free Hummus and/or some cauliflower rice.

ALMOND MEAL–CRUSTED CHICKEN FINGERS

PREP TIME: 10 MINUTES / COOK TIME: 20 MINUTES

How many of you remember being fed chicken fingers and nuggets when you were younger? How many of you remember eating chicken fingers and nuggets, um, well, a few days ago? How many of you knew that you can still eat chicken fingers while following the keto diet, with just a little alteration? I've got your back.

Nonstick cooking spray

1 cup almond meal

1 teaspoon garlic powder

½ teaspoon ground cumin

½ teaspoon paprika

¼ teaspoon cayenne pepper

2 eggs

1½ tablespoon olive oil, to brush on the fingers before basting

1 pound boneless, skinless chicken tenders

Fresh spinach leaves, for serving (optional)

Sugar-free ketchup, barbecue sauce, or sugar-free hot sauce, for serving (optional)

1. Preheat the oven to 425°F. Line a baking sheet with aluminum foil and coat with nonstick spray.

2. In a shallow bowl, combine the almond meal, garlic powder, cumin, paprika, and cayenne.

3. Crack the eggs into another shallow bowl and beat them.

4. Brush olive oil on your fingers. Working one at a time, dip the chicken tenders into the egg mixture, letting the excess drip off. Dredge in the almond meal mixture to fully coat, then place on the prepared baking sheet.

ALMOND MEAL–CRUSTED CHICKEN FINGERS *continues*

BULK COOK, SUPER QUICK

4

SERVINGS

Per Serving: Calories: 206; Total Fat: 14g; Total Carbohydrates: 3g; Net Carbs: 1g; Fiber: 2g; Protein: 17g

Macronutrients: Fat 62%; Protein 33%; Carbs 5%

SWAP: *If you cannot eat nuts, you can use coconut flour or flax meal instead.*

BRAND: *The brands of sugar-free ketchup I use regularly are Heinz, which can be found at your local grocery store, and Primal Kitchen, which can be found at Whole Foods and Sprouts. As for sugar-free bar-becue sauce, you can find G Hughes brand sugar-free barbecue sauce at Target. And, of course, you can always find these products online.*

5. Bake the chicken tenders for about 20 minutes, checking them periodically and flipping about halfway through.

6. Serve the tenders, if desired, on a bed of spinach along with some sugar-free ketchup, barbecue sauce, or hot sauce!

TIP: *These chicken tenders can be made ahead and then frozen for future use. Prep them all the way up to the cook-ing point, then place them into a freezer bag and freeze until you want a quick and easy meal. When you're ready, bake from frozen, 35 to 40 minutes in the oven or 30 minutes in an air fryer.*

MEATLOAF MUFFINS

PREP TIME: 10 MINUTES / COOK TIME: 40 MINUTES

Next time you are in charge of supplying the office kitchen or break room with food, bring these muffins. They may have your coworkers scratching their heads at first, but after one bite they will most likely dub you the Office Muffin Queen because, lady, these muffins are addictive.

Nonstick cooking spray
1 to 2 tablespoons olive oil
½ cup chopped onions
1 teaspoon garlic powder
¼ cup shredded carrots
½ cup chopped mushrooms
½ cup chopped green bell pepper
1 pound ground turkey (the fattier, the better)
1 egg
1 teaspoon dried thyme
1 teaspoon dried rosemary
1 teaspoon mustard
Sugar-free ketchup, for spreading

BULK COOK

2–4
SERVINGS
(MAKES ABOUT
9 MUFFINS)

Per Serving: Calories: 346; Total Fat: 26g; Total Carbohydrates: 6g; Net Carbs: 5g; Fiber: 1g; Protein: 22g

Macronutrients: Fat 68%; Protein 25%; Carbs 7%

1. Preheat the oven to 350°F. Coat a muffin tin with nonstick spray.

2. Heat the olive oil in a sauté pan over medium-high heat. Add the onions and season with the garlic powder. Add the carrots, mushrooms, and bell pepper and cook for 3 to 5 minutes, or until the onion is translucent.

3. Put the ground turkey in a shallow mixing bowl and add the vegetable mixture. Crack the egg on top, then add the thyme, rosemary, and mustard. Use clean hands to mix until well combined.

4. Divide the turkey mixture evenly among the cups of the prepared muffin tin and bake for about 15 minutes.

MEATLOAF MUFFINS *continues*

TRIVIA: *In ¼ cup of shredded carrots, there are about 3 grams of carbohydrates, .9 of which is from fiber, leaving 2.1 grams of net carbohydrates. If you make four muffins and only eat one, you're con-suming only .5 grams of carbohydrates from the carrots. Even though the keto diet doesn't condone eating lots of carrots, this amount will not halt ketosis.*

5. Remove the turkey muffins from the oven and slather each one with about 1 teaspoon of ketchup. Place back in the oven and bake for another 15 minutes, or until the meat is flaky and no longer pink.

6. Serve the meatloaf muffins warm out of the oven.

TIP: *If you don't have a muffin tin, you can easily make these into burgers or use a loaf pan. Know that the cooking time will need to be altered. Another tip is that these are absolutely perfect for taking on the go. Throw one or two in a zip-top bag and devour as a snack when you're hungry.*

SWAP: *If you'd prefer to use another meat, ground chicken, beef, or pork would work well for this recipe, but, as always, macronutrients and cooking times will vary.*

MEZZE CAKE

PREP TIME: 10 MINUTES / COOK TIME: 35 MINUTES

Each individual ingredient in this recipe is very attractive on its own, but caking them all together results in quite the gorgeous sight. Beyond how good it looks, you will be blown away by the sweet and savory combination that twirls together with each bite. You can serve this dish with Eggplant Chips (page 72), if you'd like.

Nonstick cooking spray

2 coconut wraps (one of them is optional)

1 small eggplant, thinly sliced lengthwise

Salt

1 zucchini, thinly sliced lengthwise

1 (8-ounce) jar sun-dried tomatoes packed in olive oil (do not discard oil), chopped or whole

½ (14-ounce) can quartered artichoke hearts

½ cup cauliflower rice

¼ cup black olives, pitted and coarsely chopped

2 precooked sugar-free chicken sausages, cut into bite-size pieces

1 tablespoon dried oregano or marjoram

½ tablespoon garlic powder

Freshly ground black pepper

BULK COOK, ONE POT

2–4
SERVINGS

Per Serving: Calories: 510; Total Fat: 38g; Total Carbohydrates: 25g; Net Carbs: 13g; Fiber: 12g; Protein: 17g

Macronutrients: Fat 67%; Protein 13%; Carbs 20%

1. Preheat the oven to 350°F. Coat a shallow baking dish with nonstick spray and place a coconut wrap in the bottom.

2. Sprinkle the eggplant with ½ teaspoon of salt and let sit for 5 minutes to let the moisture come to the surface. Get a damp towel and wipe off the salt and excess water from the eggplant.

MEZZE CAKE *continues*

SWAP: *Omit the meat and add 2 or 3 eggs or about 8 ounces of firm tofu if you want a vegetarian version of this dish.*

TRIVIA: *Artichokes contain phytochemicals called cynarine and silymarin that have been touted for their ability to aid in liver health. A healthy liver is of the utmost importance as it filters blood, detoxifies our bodies from harmful chemicals, and makes proteins that help blood clot.*

3. Lay the eggplant slices on top of the coconut wrap, then lay the zucchini slices on top of the eggplant. Next add the sun-dried tomatoes and drizzle in the olive oil they're packed in. Sprinkle in the artichoke hearts, then add the cauliflower rice. Scatter the olives on top, then shower the chicken sausage over all the vegetables. Season everything with the oregano, garlic powder, salt, and pepper.

4. Place another coconut wrap over the top of everything, if desired, and bake this vegetable layer "cake" in the oven for about 25 minutes, or until the vegetables are a bit wilted.

5. Turn the oven to broil and cook for another 5 minutes, or until the top is crisp.

6. Remove from the oven and let cool before slicing and serving.

TIP: *If you have extra Breakfast Sausage (page 58) on hand, you can use that in this recipe instead of the chicken sausage.*

AVOCADO "TOAST"

PREP TIME: 10 MINUTES / COOK TIME: 20 MINUTES

Remember when avocado toast took the world by storm? Well, I took matters into my own hands and made a version of avocado toast that satisfies the craving yet isn't even toast at all. Ground turkey takes the place of the glucose-spiking grain. Perhaps this high-protein, high-fat rendition will be the next "it" food combo.

1 tablespoon avocado oil or nonstick cooking spray

8 ounces ground turkey (50 percent dark meat, 50 percent light meat)

½ teaspoon dried thyme

½ teaspoon dried rosemary

½ teaspoon dried sage

¼ teaspoon garlic powder

½ teaspoon freshly ground black pepper, plus more for seasoning

¼ teaspoon paprika

¼ teaspoon salt, plus more for seasoning

1 small avocado, halved and pitted

Freshly squeezed lime juice (optional)

"Everything bagel" spice, for serving (optional)

Cherry tomatoes, halved, for serving (optional)

SUPER QUICK

1-2
SERVINGS

Per Serving: Calories: 466; Total Fat: 38g; Total Carbohydrates: 9g; Net Carbs: 3g; Fiber: 6g; Protein: 22g

Macronutrients: Fat 73%; Protein 19%; Carbs 8%

1. Preheat the oven to 400°F. Coat a baking sheet with the avocado oil or nonstick spray.

2. In a large mixing bowl, combine the ground turkey with the thyme, rosemary, sage, garlic powder, pepper, paprika, and salt. Using clean hands, mix everything together until well combined.

3. Dump the ground turkey mixture onto the prepared baking sheet and press as flat as you can. Bake for about 20 minutes, flipping halfway through, until the meat is flaky and no longer pink.

AVOCADO "TOAST" *continues*

SWAP: *If you're not a fan of the spices used in this recipe, feel free to use any you prefer.*

4. Meanwhile, scoop the avocado flesh into a separate mixing bowl, season with salt, pepper, and a squeeze of lime juice (if using), and mash with a fork until smooth.

5. Remove the turkey from the oven and, when cool enough to handle, use a knife to cut it into toast-like squares.

6. Spread the mashed avocado over the top of the turkey "toast" and, if desired, serve seasoned with "everything bagel" spice and topped with halved cherry tomatoes.

TIP: *Determine if an avocado is ripe by removing the stem and observing the color underneath. If it's green, the avocado is ripe. If it's black or very dark brown, it's overripe. If the stem doesn't come off at all, then it's not ripe yet.*

TURKEY-STUFFED AVOCADOS

PREP TIME: 5 TO 10 MINUTES / COOK TIME: 5 TO 10 MINUTES

Eating the same thing day after day can get boring, and when you roast a whole turkey, you may wind up eating leftovers for three or four days. Instead of reheating the turkey, which can dry it out, this recipe will help liven up the meat's taste and texture and have you thinking you're eating a whole new meal, even though it takes no time to make.

4 asparagus spears, trimmed

1½ cups cubed roasted turkey

2 cups fresh spinach, chopped

¼ cup avocado oil mayonnaise

Salt

Freshly ground black pepper

2 large avocados, halved and pitted

1. Fill a pot with ¼ inch of water and bring to a boil over medium-high heat. Add the asparagus, cover, and cook for 5 to 10 minutes, until tender (or to your desired doneness).

2. Meanwhile, in a mixing bowl, combine the turkey with the spinach and mayonnaise and season with salt and pepper.

3. When the asparagus is done, remove from the pot, chop into pieces, and add it to the bowl with the turkey. Mix until everything is evenly coated with the mayonnaise.

4. If the cavities in your avocados where the pits were are big enough, spoon in the turkey mixture and serve. If the cavities are not big enough, scoop out some of the avocado flesh and mix into the turkey mixture before spooning into the cavities.

TIP: *If you have turkey mixture left over, it makes for the perfect snack or a wonderful meal on the go.*

SUPER QUICK

2-4
SERVINGS

Per Serving: Calories: 624; Total Fat: 48g; Total Carbohydrates: 17g; Net Carbs: 4g; Fiber: 13g; Protein: 31g

Macronutrients: Fat 70%; Protein 20%; Carbs 10%

SWAP: *You can easily swap in hard-boiled eggs or chicken for the turkey.*

CHICKEN FAJITAS

PREP TIME: 10 MINUTES / COOK TIME: 15 TO 20 MINUTES

When you make fajitas at home, you have complete control of all the ingredients and the ability to make them keto-approved. And if you want a little of the sweetness that your local joint might include in their spice mix, the cinnamon found in this recipe, known to regulate blood sugar, will help you achieve just that.

BULK COOK, SUPER QUICK

4
SERVINGS

Per Serving: Calories: 235; Total Fat: 13g; Total Carbohydrates: 5g; Net Carbs: 3g; Fiber: 2g; Protein: 25g

Macronutrients: Fat 50%; Protein 43%; Carbs 7%

1 pound boneless, skinless chicken breasts and/or thighs, sliced into thin strips

1 teaspoon salt

1 teaspoon dried oregano

1 teaspoon garlic powder

½ teaspoon freshly ground black pepper

1 teaspoon ground cumin

½ teaspoon red pepper flakes

½ teaspoon paprika

¼ teaspoon ground cinnamon

2 tablespoons avocado oil or butter, divided

½ white onion, sliced

½ red bell pepper, sliced into strips

½ green bell pepper, sliced into strips

2 tablespoons chicken broth (optional)

2 to 4 coconut or almond flour wraps, or grain-free chips

1 cup shredded romaine lettuce

Sugar-free salsa, Guacamole (page 210), sour cream, and shredded cheese, for serving (optional)

1. In a large bowl, combine the chicken with the salt, oregano, garlic powder, pepper, cumin, red pepper flakes, paprika, cinnamon, and 1 tablespoon of oil or butter.

2. Heat the remaining tablespoon of oil or butter in a large, shallow skillet over medium-high heat. Add the onion and cook for 3 to 5 minutes, stirring occasionally, until translucent.

3. Add the bell peppers and continue to cook, stirring, for another 5 minutes, until tender.

4. Add the chicken mixture and continue to cook and stir for another 2 to 3 minutes, then reduce the heat to medium, cover, and cook for about 5 minutes, or until the chicken is cooked through and no longer pink. If the chicken starts to burn, add the chicken broth.

5. Remove the chicken mixture from the heat and let cool a bit.

6. Divide the wraps or chips among plates, sprinkle the shredded romaine on top, and spoon the chicken fajita mixture on top of the lettuce. Serve the fajitas with salsa, Guacamole, sour cream, and cheese, if you'd like.

TIP: *You can buy frozen bags of sliced bell peppers and onions, so you don't have to go through the task of slicing them up yourself.*

SWAP: *If you don't have coconut or almond wraps on hand, romaine lettuce leaves are the perfect crunchy substitute with far fewer calories and carbohydrates.*

TRIVIA: *Do you know about coconut or almond flour wraps? If not, I am about to blow your mind, because you get to eat wraps again. While coconut wraps are typically made with coconut meat, water, and oil, almond flour wraps sometimes contain tapioca flour, which does have a fair amount of carbohydrates, so make sure to read labels.*

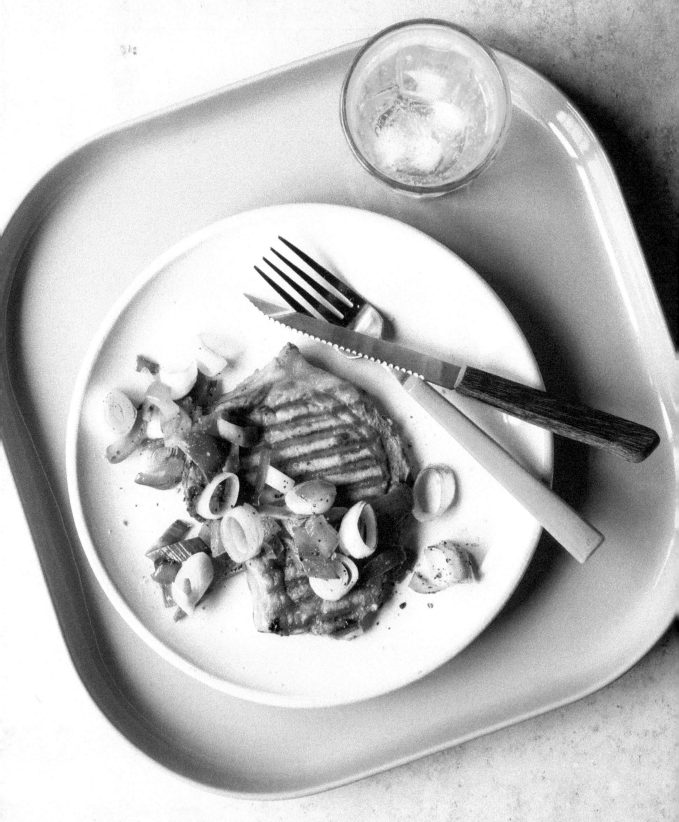

Pork Chops Smothered in Caramelized Onions & Leeks, page 177

Chapter 8

Beef & Pork

Hopefully you will love "meating" this next section of recipes, because there is no reason to shun beef and pork since they are powerhouses for essential vitamins, minerals, and amino acids—all great for a woman's overall health!

Beef & Broccoli Pizza **148**

Ground Beef Cauli-Fried Rice **150**

Meatza **152**

Cottage Pie Muffins **153**

Brisket Nachos **155**

Grilled Steak with Chimichurri **157**

Pork Tacos/Burrito Wraps **158**

Chorizo Sliders **160**

Tandoori Beef Fajitas **162**

Pork Spring Rolls **164**

Stuffed Bell Peppers **166**

Pork Pho with Shirataki Noodles **168**

Spaghetti Squash & Ground Pork Stir-Fry with Kale **170**

Beef Burgers with Bacon **172**

Slow-Cooked Shredded Beef **174**

Beef Stroganoff **175**

Pork Chops Smothered in Caramelized Onions & Leeks **177**

BEEF & BROCCOLI PIZZA

PREP TIME: 15 MINUTES / COOK TIME: 30 MINUTES

This pizza can be totally customized to your preferences. I encourage you to put on your chef's apron and think outside of the box. While this recipe is chock-full of flavorful Mediterranean goodness, you could certainly change up the taste however you'd like! And the use of dairy products is optional because nutritional yeast serves up a cheesy flavor that's totally vegan yet contains all nine essential amino acids, making it a complete protein. You can serve this pizza with Chopped Bitter Greens Salad (page 89), if you like.

3
SERVINGS

Per Serving: Calories: 428;
Total Fat: 25g; Total
Carbohydrates: 27g; Net
Carbs: 12g; Fiber: 15g;
Protein: 23g

Macronutrients: Fat 54%;
Protein 21%; Carbs 25%

1 tablespoon avocado oil or nonstick cooking spray

1 recipe French Toast bread dough (prepared through step 2 on page 56)

1 tablespoon nutritional yeast or grated cheese

½ teaspoon dried oregano

½ teaspoon garlic powder

¼ teaspoon salt

¼ teaspoon freshly ground black pepper

2 tablespoons no-sugar-added tomato sauce

6 ounces crumbled uncooked ground beef or crumbled uncooked Breakfast Sausage (page 58)

½ cup broccoli, chopped into bite-size pieces

Diced white onion, for topping (optional)

Chopped pitted olives, for topping (optional)

Shredded cheese, for topping (optional)

1 tablespoon olive oil

1. Preheat the oven to 400°F. Grease a baking sheet with avocado oil or nonstick spray.

2. To the French toast bread dough, add the nutritional yeast or grated cheese, the oregano, garlic powder, salt, and pepper.

3. Transfer the dough to the prepared baking sheet and form into a pizza-crust-like shape. Bake for 15 to 20 minutes, checking periodically, until slightly browned.

4. Remove the crust from the oven, then slather the tomato sauce all over it, leaving a ½-inch border. Sprinkle with the crumbled meat, the broccoli and, if desired, diced onion, chopped olives, and shredded cheese. Drizzle all over with the olive oil.

5. Return the pizza to the oven and bake for 5 to 6 minutes, or until the vegetables look nicely caramelized and slightly charred.

6. Remove the pizza from the oven, let cool for a minute or two, slice, and serve.

TIP: *This crust freezes very well. Feel free to make a bunch of bread or crusts in advance and freeze them for future use.*

SWAP: *Not a fan of broccoli? Use Brussels sprouts or asparagus instead. Just steam them for 3 to 5 minutes before using to top the pizza.*

GROUND BEEF CAULI-FRIED RICE

PREP TIME: 5 TO 10 MINUTES / COOK TIME: 15 TO 20 MINUTES

Who eats just one serving of fried rice? Not me! Thankfully you can chow down on this scrumptious dish as long as you use riced cauliflower in place of white rice. To further improve the nutritional quality, using grass-fed and -finished beef will amp up the omega-3 fatty acids. Plus, by making your favorite fast food at home, you slash the calories and the unnecessary ingredients, which aids your body in becoming a keto powerhouse!

**BULK COOK,
ONE POT,
SUPER QUICK**

1-2
SERVINGS

Per Serving: Calories: 502;
Total Fat: 34g; Total
Carbohydrates: 17g; Net Carbs:
10g; Fiber: 7g; Protein: 32g

Macronutrients: Fat 62%;
Protein 25%; Carbs 13%

1 tablespoon avocado or sesame oil

6 asparagus spears, trimmed and finely chopped

5 scallions, finely chopped

1 (12-ounce) bag frozen cauliflower rice

1 cup Bone Broth (page 203)

1 egg

½ pound 80% lean ground beef

1 tablespoon tamari or coconut aminos

1 teaspoon minced pickled ginger

Garlic powder

Fresh spinach leaves or Asian Cucumber Salad (page 94),
   for serving (optional)

1. Heat the oil in a shallow skillet or wok over medium-high heat. Add the asparagus and scallions and cook for 2 to 3 minutes.

2. Add the frozen cauliflower rice, stir everything together, and cook for another 3 to 5 minutes.

3. Pour the Bone Broth into the skillet, then crack the egg into the skillet. Stir the entire contents of the pan together.

4. Crumble in the ground beef and stir to blend with the rest of the ingredients. Cook for 3 to 5 minutes, or until the meat is browned.

5. Season with the tamari, ginger, and garlic powder to taste, then stir and cook for another 3 minutes.

6. Serve on a bed of spinach or with cucumber salad.

TIP: *Pickled ginger makes this recipe's flavor wonderfully pungent—it's even better than using powdered or grated ginger from the root.*

SWAP: *If you're sick of using cauliflower as a grain replacement, you can use riced butternut squash or riced broccoli.*

TRIVIA: *Bone broth has been shown to have numerous health benefits, including as an aid in the treatment of leaky gut syndrome. It also improves joint health, reduces the appearance of cellulite, and boosts the immune system.*

MEATZA

PREP TIME: 5 TO 10 MINUTES / COOK TIME: 25 MINUTES

Who's willing to give up Friday night pizza? You don't have to as long as you make your pizza meaty—as in, the crust is made out of meat. Meat doesn't spike your insulin levels nearly as much as carbohydrates!

1-2
SERVINGS

Per Serving: Calories: 349; Total Fat: 21g; Total Carbohydrates: 15g; Net Carbs: 9g; Fiber: 6g; Protein: 25g

Macronutrients: Fat 55%; Protein 29%; Carbs 16%

TIP: *Depending on the percentage of fat your ground beef has—the fattier the better in my opinion—it can be greasy. This can lead to intense bubbling, so be careful when removing it from the oven.*

SWAP: *You can substitute ground pork, turkey, or chicken, or even use eggs to make the crust.*

2 tablespoons avocado oil, divided
½ pound ground beef
½ cup cauliflower rice
¼ cup minced carrots
Salt
Freshly ground black pepper
3 tablespoons no-sugar-added tomato sauce
2 tablespoons chopped white onion
Chopped zucchini, eggplant, or leeks, for topping (optional)
Shredded cheese, for topping (optional)
Roasted Brussels sprouts or sliced avocado, for serving

1. Preheat the oven to 360°F. Line a baking sheet with aluminum foil and grease with 1 tablespoon of oil.

2. In a mixing bowl, combine the ground beef, cauliflower, and carrots. Season with salt and pepper. Use clean hands to mix together until well combined.

3. Transfer the meat mixture to the prepared baking sheet and press into a round pizza shape. Bake for 10 to 12 minutes, until the meat is browned.

4. Take the meat crust out of the oven, then slather the tomato sauce all over it, leaving a ½-inch border. Sprinkle with the onion, any other chopped veggies you'd like, and shredded cheese if you want.

5. Put the meatza back in the oven and cook for another 10 minutes, until the vegetables are crisp.

6. Remove from the oven and let cool before slicing and serving with Brussels sprouts or avocado.

COTTAGE PIE MUFFINS

PREP TIME: 10 MINUTES / COOK TIME: 35 TO 40 MINUTES

Let's get to the meat and potatoes here. Well, the meat, anyway. Cottage pie is a savory pie typically comprised of a meaty mixture topped with mashed potatoes. In this recipe, the potatoes have been replaced with cauliflower, giving you a texture and flavor similar to potatoes with far fewer carbs. This dish is full of bold and comforting flavors and ingredients that you will certainly want to savor.

2 tablespoons coconut oil, divided

½ medium onion, diced

1 cup diced cremini mushrooms

½ cup diced celery

¼ cup diced carrot

Salt

Freshly ground black pepper

1 pound ground free-range pork or wild boar

½ teaspoon garlic powder

½ teaspoon dried oregano

½ teaspoon dried thyme

½ head cauliflower, chopped into bite-size florets

½ cup Bone Broth (page 203)

1 tablespoon full-fat coconut milk or regular milk (optional)

Shredded Irish Cheddar cheese (optional)

Chopped fresh tarragon or dill, for serving (optional)

BULK COOK

2-4
SERVINGS

Per Serving: Calories: 266; Total Fat: 18g; Total Carbohydrates: 3g; Net Carbs: 2g; Fiber: 1g; Protein: 23g

Macronutrients: Fat 61%; Protein 35%; Carbs 4%

1. Preheat the oven to 380°F. Coat a muffin tin with 1 tablespoon of coconut oil (alternatively, you can line the muffin cups with muffin cup liners).

2. In a shallow sauté pan, heat the remaining 1 tablespoon of coconut oil over medium-high heat. Add the onion, mushrooms, celery, and carrot, season with salt and pepper, and cook for about 10 minutes, stirring occasionally, until the veggies are a bit limp.

COTTAGE PIE MUFFINS *continues*

TIP: *If made in a muffin tin, these little pies are perfect for on-the-go meals. Just put one or two in a plastic bag and you're all set.*

SWAP: *Instead of cauliflower as the topping, you can use puréed pumpkin. Leave out the bone broth and add 1 to 2 tablespoons of coconut or almond flour to thicken the purée.*

3. Crumble the ground meat into the pan and season with the garlic powder, oregano, and thyme. Stir everything together and cook for 3 to 5 minutes.

4. Transfer the meat and vegetable mixture to a bowl and let rest while you prepare the cauliflower.

5. In a pot over medium-high heat, bring ¼ inch of water to a boil. Add the cauliflower and steam for 3 to 4 minutes.

6. Drain the cauliflower and transfer to a blender along with the bone broth. Blend until it has reached a creamy, smooth texture. Add the milk to the mix if needed to reach that consistency.

7. Fill the prepared muffin tin with the meat and vegetable mixture. Use a spatula or spoon to "frost" the muffins with the puréed cauliflower. Season with salt and pepper and bake in the oven for about 15 minutes, sprinkling with cheese (if using) in the last 5 minutes or so. The muffins are done when the top has formed a crust and the cheese is oozy.

8. Remove the muffins from the oven and let cool, then sprinkle with dill or tarragon (if using) and chow down!

BRISKET NACHOS

PREP TIME: 20 MINUTES / COOK TIME: 2 HOURS

In place of traditional chips that are high in carbohydrates, this recipe calls for roasted or air-fried celery root, rutabaga, or turnip. It also skips the beans, which drive up the carb count, and leaves out the ground meat. Instead, this recipe swaps in what some barbecue lovers might call the crème de la crème of any barbecue offering: juicy, tender brisket. Brisket might sound intimidating to make, but it's worth every second of preparation and cook time. With this recipe, you'll be a master in no time.

1 pound beef brisket

3 tablespoons avocado oil, divided

1½ teaspoons red pepper flakes

1½ teaspoons salt, plus more for seasoning

1½ teaspoons garlic powder

1½ teaspoons onion powder

1½ teaspoons erythritol "brown sugar"

1 teaspoon freshly ground black pepper, plus more for seasoning

1 teaspoon mustard

¾ cup Bone Broth (page 203)

1 medium celery root, or rutabaga, sliced into ¼-inch-thick rounds

1 medium onion, sliced into strips

Fresh spinach leaves, for serving (optional)

Sugar-free barbecue sauce, shredded Cheddar cheese, and diced avocado, for topping (optional)

4

SERVINGS

Per Serving: Calories: 326; Total Fat: 22g; Total Carbohydrates: 7g; Net Carbs: 5g; Fiber: 2g; Protein: 25g; Erythritol: 2g

Macronutrients: Fat 61%; Protein 30%; Carbs 9%

1. Preheat the oven to 350°F.

2. Rub the brisket all over with 1 tablespoon of avocado oil and season on both sides with the red pepper flakes, salt, garlic powder, onion powder, erythritol, pepper, and mustard.

3. Place the meat in a roasting pan with a rack and roast for 30 minutes.

BRISKET NACHOS *continues*

TIP: *I recommend eating this meal the same day you cook it. These nachos don't keep very well because the brisket's fat will make the chips soggy.*

SWAP: *If you're short on time, you can, of course, make this recipe with ground beef or pork.*

BRAND: *US Wellness Meats, an online retailer, has precooked, sugar-free smoked and sliced brisket available for sale. It's absolutely delicious and works perfectly for this recipe, saving you time and energy.*

4. Remove the brisket from the oven and add the bone broth. Cover with aluminum foil, return to the oven, and continue to roast for 1 hour and 30 minutes, or until the meat is fork-tender.

5. Meanwhile, make your "chips." Put the celery root on a baking dish and rub with 1 tablespoon of avocado oil. Roast in the oven for about 35 minutes, turning once, until browned on both sides. Alternatively, you can cook them in an air fryer for 30 minutes, stirring once or twice, until browned all over.

6. When the brisket has about 10 minutes left to cook, in a shallow skillet, heat the remaining 1 tablespoon of avocado oil over medium-high heat. Add the onion and sauté for about 5 minutes, or until translucent. Add a little salt to the pan to bring out the onion's sweetness.

7. Remove the brisket from the oven and slice into thin strips. Put the vegetable chips on a serving plate. Top with some spinach leaves (if using) and the brisket. If desired, drizzle with barbecue sauce and sprinkle with cheese and diced avocado.

GRILLED STEAK WITH CHIMICHURRI

PREP TIME: 10 MINUTES / COOK TIME: 20 MINUTES

Parsley is typically thought of as a garnish, but it's full of calcium, iron, vitamin A, and chemical compounds that can encourage menstruation. Parsley plays the starring role in this delicious recipe, with its flavor pairing amazingly well with the steak cut of your choice.

¾ cup chopped fresh parsley

½ cup avocado or olive oil, plus 1 tablespoon

1 tablespoon balsamic vinegar

4 garlic cloves, coarsely chopped

1 tablespoon dried marjoram

1 tablespoon dried oregano

2 teaspoons red pepper flakes

Salt

Freshly ground black pepper

2 (6-ounce) steaks (beef, lamb, elk, venison, or bison)

Cooked cauliflower or Cauliflower "Potato" Salad (page 95), for serving

1. In a food processor or blender, combine the parsley, ½ cup of oil, the vinegar, garlic, marjoram, oregano, red pepper flakes, salt, and pepper together until smooth.

2. Slather a grill with the remaining 1 tablespoon of oil and then preheat. Alternatively, heat the tablespoon of oil in a shallow sauté pan over medium-high heat.

3. Throw the steaks on the grill or add to the sauté pan and cook to your desired doneness, 3 to 5 minutes per side for medium-rare. (I personally like my meat very rare, so I would cook for 2 to 3 minutes per side.)

4. Serve the steak drizzled with the chimichurri sauce, with cooked cauliflower or Cauliflower "Potato" Salad on the side.

BULK COOK, SUPER QUICK

2
SERVINGS

Per Serving: Calories: 790; Total Fat: 68g; Total Carbohydrates: 7g; Net Carbs: 4g; Fiber: 3g; Protein: 40g

Macronutrients: Fat 69%; Protein 21%; Carbs 10%

SWAP: *Make the chimichurri with flax oil, instead of avocado or olive oil, to give it a nuttier flavor. Keep in mind that flax oil must be refrigerated and should never be cooked.*

PORK TACOS/BURRITO WRAPS

PREP TIME: 5 TO 10 MINUTES (PLUS AT LEAST 30 MINUTES OF MARINATING TIME) / COOK TIME: 15 TO 20 MINUTES

Making this pork taco or burrito takes next to no time because all you need to do is combine the seasonings listed and pour them over hunks of pork tenderloin, cook for about 15 minutes, wrap everything up, and enjoy. I've always been a believer that home-cooked meals should be dubbed the real "fast food." Hopefully, this recipe, along with many others found in this book, will have you thinking the same thing! This dish is great for when you have a few people over because your guests can prepare their tacos however they choose. Of course, when eating tacos or burritos, it's important to have a Virgin (or Not) Mojito (page 202) to accompany the tasty meal.

4-6
SERVINGS

Per Serving: Calories: 640; Total Fat: 44g; Total Carbohydrates: 26g; Net Carbs: 14g; Fiber: 12g; Protein: 35g

Macronutrients: Fat 62%; Protein 22%; Carbs 16%

3 tablespoons avocado oil, divided

5 tablespoons chopped fresh cilantro, divided

½ teaspoon dried oregano

¼ teaspoon ground cinnamon

¼ teaspoon allspice

½ teaspoon paprika

½ teaspoon garlic powder

½ teaspoon onion powder

1 tablespoon chili powder

¼ teaspoon salt

¼ teaspoon white pepper

1½ pounds pork tenderloin, cut into ½-inch cubes

4 to 6 coconut flour or jicama wraps

1 small head lettuce, shredded

1 small white onion, sliced

Guacamole (page 210), sugar-free salsa, sour cream, shredded cheese, and lime wedges, for serving (optional)

1. In a large resealable plastic bag, combine 2 tablespoons of avocado oil with 3 tablespoons of cilantro, the oregano, cinnamon, allspice, paprika, garlic, onion, and chili powders, salt, and white pepper. Add the pork cubes to the bag, seal tightly, and then shake to evenly coat the meat in the marinade. Marinate in the refrigerator for at least 30 minutes or up to 24 hours.

2. Take the meat out of the refrigerator and let it come to room temperature.

3. Heat the remaining 1 tablespoon of oil in a shallow skillet over medium-high heat. Toss the pork into the pan along with its marinade juices and cook for about 15 minutes, until it is crumbly and no longer pink.

4. To serve, lay the wraps on plates and top each with some of the lettuce and onion slices. Scoop the pork on top and garnish with the remaining 2 tablespoons of cilantro. If you'd like, finish off with Guacamole, salsa, sour cream, and/or cheese, with lime wedges on the side for squeezing. Fold up into a taco or roll up into a burrito and enjoy.

TIP: *If you make extra, you can have a taco salad for lunch or dinner the following day.*

SWAP: *This recipe can easily be made with ground pork or any beef cut you'd like.*

CHORIZO SLIDERS

PREP TIME: 15 MINUTES / COOK TIME: 25 MINUTES

Go on, slide these sliders into your mouth, and, yes, you can eat more than one! These little burgers are perfect as an elaborate breakfast recipe, a tasty snack, or even a crowd-pleasing appetizer if you're hosting a party—that is, if you're willing to share!

BULK COOK

2
SERVINGS

Per Serving: Calories: 734;
Total Fat: 50g; Total
Carbohydrates: 24g; Net
Carbs: 16g; Fiber: 8g;
Protein: 47g

Macronutrients: Fat 61%;
Protein 26%; Carbs 13%

8 small portobello mushroom caps

2 tablespoons avocado oil or butter, divided

Salt

Freshly ground black pepper

1 recipe uncooked Breakfast Sausage (made with pork; page 58)

4 butter lettuce leaves

4 red onion slices

4 plum tomato slices

4 slices grass-fed/-finished pepper Jack cheese (optional)

Sugar-free pickles, sugar-free ketchup, mustard, sugar-free barbecue sauce, and/or cooked bacon, for serving (optional)

Chipotle-lime mayonnaise, for spreading (optional)

1. Preheat the oven to 350°F.

2. Wipe the mushroom caps off with a damp towel and then place them on a baking sheet. Brush them with 1 tablespoon of oil or butter, then season with salt and pepper. Roast in the oven for 15 to 20 minutes, or until browned and crispy.

3. When the mushrooms have about 10 minutes left to cook, form the uncooked sausage meat into four slider-size burger patties.

4. Heat the remaining 1 tablespoon of oil in a shallow skillet over medium-high heat and cook the burger patties for about 5 minutes per side, or until completely cooked through.

5. Place 4 mushrooms cap-side down on plates. Place a piece of butter lettuce on each mushroom, then slide a burger onto each piece of lettuce.

6. Top the sliders with the onion and tomato, then feel free to add a slice of cheese and top with pickles, ketchup, mustard, barbecue sauce, and/or crispy bacon. Slather a little chipotle mayonnaise on the other 4 mushroom caps, if you'd like, close the sliders, and serve. (If serving at a party, you can use toothpicks to hold the sliders together.)

TIP: *You can make your ground pork patties smaller to yield more sliders, but you will need to use more portobello mushroom caps or serve your sliders open-face.*

SWAP: *If you aren't a fan of mushrooms, use Eggplant Chips (page 72) for the buns instead. Just cut the eggplant into thicker slices to be more bun-like.*

BRAND: *Mt. Olive and Vlasic sell sugar-free pickles on Amazon.com. Heinz sells sugar-free ketchup, which can be found at your local grocery store or on Amazon.com. G Hughes has a line of sugar-free barbecue sauce that can be purchased online, and Primal Kitchen offers up a delicious chipotle-lime mayonnaise made with avocado oil.*

TANDOORI BEEF FAJITAS

PREP TIME: 5 TO 10 MINUTES (PLUS 2 TO 24 HOURS MARINATING TIME) /
COOK TIME: 10 TO 15 MINUTES

Let's mix and match flavors and cooking methods, shall we? Tandoori is an Indian marinade, typically used for chicken, but I am breaking the rules and using it on beef in this recipe, then cooking it fajita-style, which is a technique native to Mexico!

BULK COOK

2
SERVINGS

Per Serving: Calories: 655; Total Fat: 43g; Total Carbohydrates: 16g; Net Carbs: 12g; Fiber: 4g; Protein: 51g

Macronutrients: Fat 60%; Protein 30%; Carbs 10%

½ cup sugar-free, grass-fed/-finished Greek yogurt (optional)

2 tablespoons avocado oil

½ teaspoon garlic powder

½ teaspoon ground cumin

½ teaspoon paprika

½ teaspoon ground coriander

¼ teaspoon ground cinnamon

¼ teaspoon ground turmeric

¼ teaspoon cayenne pepper

¼ teaspoon ground ginger

¼ teaspoon erythritol "brown sugar"

Salt

1 pound sirloin or flank steak, sliced into strips

1 tablespoon grass-fed/-finished butter or butter-flavored coconut oil

2 medium bell peppers (any color), sliced

1 medium red onion, sliced

4 ounces button mushrooms, sliced (optional)

8 asparagus spears, trimmed and chopped (optional)

2 to 4 coconut or almond flour wraps or grain-free chips

1 cup shredded romaine lettuce

Sugar-free salsa, sour cream, Guacamole (page 210), and shredded cheese, for serving (optional)

1. In a large resealable plastic bag, combine the Greek yogurt (if using), avocado oil, garlic, cumin, paprika, coriander, cinnamon, turmeric, cayenne, ginger, erythritol and salt. Add the steak, seal the bag tightly, and massage the marinade into the meat until it is well coated. Marinate in the refrigerator for at least 2 hours or up to 24 hours. (You can marinate it for less than 2 hours if you'd like, but I personally think marinating for longer makes a difference in flavor.)

2. In a shallow sauté pan or wok over medium-high heat, melt the butter or coconut oil. Add the bell peppers, onion, mushrooms (if using), and asparagus (if using) to the pan and cook for 5 to 8 minutes, or until the onion is translucent and the vegetables are tender.

3. Meanwhile, remove the beef from the marinade and transfer to a cutting board (don't discard the marinade).

4. Toss the strips of beef into the pan and pour in the remaining marinade from the bag. Stir-fry everything together for 5 to 8 minutes, or until the meat is cooked through to your liking. Be sure the marinade boils for at least 1 full minute to kill off any harmful bacteria.

5. Place the wraps or chips on plates and top with shredded lettuce. Top with the beef fajita mixture, then dole up some salsa, sour cream, Guacamole, and cheese however you please (if using).

TIP: *If you like your food extremely spicy, increase the amount of cayenne pepper in this recipe.*

SWAP: *If you don't have all of the herbs and spices required for this recipe, you can purchase a premade mixture; just make sure it's 100 percent sugar-free. Patak's Original tandoori marinade is an option. Frontier Co-Op also has a tandoori masala seasoning that would work perfectly, as well.*

BRAND: *The Real Coconut has some of the best keto-approved chips I have ever tasted. Stick to recommended serving sizes because you can easily consume way too many carbohydrates if you don't pay attention. For a much lower carbohydrate alternative that still gives you the crunch, pork rinds are the way to go. Just make sure they're sugar-free and free-range.*

PORK SPRING ROLLS

PREP TIME: 15 MINUTES / COOK TIME: 15 TO 20 MINUTES

Years ago, when I traveled to Vietnam with my family, we took a cooking class and roamed the streets for hours, weaving in and out of food markets. The person leading our class introduced us to many foods we had never heard of while picking up every ingredient necessary for the dishes we would be making. We learned the Vietnamese culinary basics in a small, hot room where we wound up creating culinary witchcraft. Included in this sorcery were pork spring rolls, which will forever be a fond memory for my taste buds. Thanks to that memory, I was able to create a keto-approved spring roll recipe, which may have you saying "abracadabra" after your first bite.

1-2
SERVINGS

Per Serving: Calories: 513; Total Fat: 33g; Total Carbohydrates: 27g; Net Carbs: 13g; Fiber: 14g; Protein: 27g

Macronutrients: Fat 60%; Protein 20%; Carbs 20%

2½ tablespoons avocado oil, divided

½ pound ground free-range pork or wild boar

½ medium jicama, peeled and grated

1 small carrot, peeled and grated

1 small summer squash, grated

1½ cups fresh spinach, coarsely chopped

2½ tablespoons pickled ginger, finely chopped

1 egg

Salt

Freshly ground black pepper

2 coconut flour wraps

Yum Yum Sauce (page 217), coconut aminos, or tamari, for dipping (optional)

1. In a shallow skillet, heat 1¼ tablespoons of avocado oil over medium-high heat. Add the ground meat and cook until absolutely no pink is visible, 8 to 10 minutes. Transfer to a mixing bowl.

2. Add the jicama, carrot, summer squash, spinach, and pickled ginger to the bowl. Crack in the egg, season with salt and pepper, and mix everything together.

3. Lay the wraps on a work surface or cutting board and brush them with a little bit of water to make them pliable. Place about half of the meat mixture on one side of each wrap and fold up like a burrito.

4. In a shallow skillet (use the same one as before), heat the remaining 1¼ tablespoons of avocado oil over medium-high heat. Add the spring rolls and fry on each side for 3 to 5 minutes, or until the wraps start to char and are nicely crisped.

5. You can eat these spring rolls plain or serve them with dipping sauce.

TIP: *If you've had to buy a whole pound of meat for this recipe, use the other half pound to make Breakfast Sausage (page 58) the next morning. If you have leftover jicama, swap it for the cauliflower in the Breakfast Bowl (page 59) to make jicama hash.*

SWAP: *You can air-fry these spring rolls instead of pan-frying. This will reduce the fat used in the recipe, so beware that you may need to eat more fat in another meal in order to balance out your macronutrient intake for the day.*

STUFFED BELL PEPPERS

PREP TIME: 5 TO 10 MINUTES / COOK TIME: 45 MINUTES

Bell peppers are totally the purses of the produce world. I know, it's a weird idea, but think about it: They can hold anything you'd like, much like your purse! This recipe includes so many flavorful ingredients, you'll want to stuff as much into this veggie purse as possible. Unlike searching through your real purse, though, which sometimes feels like a black hole, you will always find what you're looking for with these because you can see all the ingredients without having to dig!

4
SERVINGS

Per Serving: Calories: 378;
Total Fat: 26g; Total
Carbohydrates: 14g;
Net Carbs: 11g; Fiber: 3g;
Protein: 22g

Macronutrients: Fat 62%;
Protein 23%; Carbs 15%

4 bell peppers (any color)

½ pound 80% lean ground beef

½ pound ground free-range pork

½ large onion, chopped

½ tablespoon garlic powder

2 teaspoons dried basil

¾ cup canned tomato sauce or jarred sugar-free tomato sauce

½ cup shredded cheese or nutritional yeast, plus more for serving (optional)

Chopped fresh basil (optional)

1. Preheat the oven to 350°F.
2. Chop off the tops of the bell peppers and remove the seeds and ribs.
3. In a shallow skillet over medium-high heat, cook the beef and pork along with the onion, garlic powder, and dried basil for 3 to 5 minutes, or until the meat is browned.
4. Add the tomato sauce and cheese (or nutritional yeast) and stir until everything is combined.
5. Fill the cavity of each bell pepper with the mixture, then place each stuffed pepper in a baking dish. Cover with aluminum foil and roast in the oven for about 30 minutes.

6. Remove the foil and check to make sure the peppers are roasting nicely, then cook, uncovered, for another 10 minutes, or until the peppers are slightly charred and the filling is crisp.

7. Transfer the stuffed peppers to plates and lightly sprinkle with fresh basil, if desired. Feel free to top with more cheese or nutritional yeast if you'd like.

TIP: *If you have leftover stuffing mixture, don't fret. Save it to top leafy greens or scramble it with eggs for breakfast the next day.*

SWAP: *To get the traditional texture of rice in your peppers, add cauliflower rice or broccoli to the skillet when you brown the meat.*

PORK PHO WITH SHIRATAKI NOODLES

PREP TIME: 15 MINUTES / COOK TIME: 1 HOUR

You may have thought pho, the delicious Vietnamese soup that typically consists of rice noodles, to be completely off limits while following the keto diet. However, with one simple tweak, slurping down this soup is totally possible. Swap out the rice noodles for a lower-carb replacement: shirataki noodles. These "noodles" are made from an herb native to Asia that is 97 percent water and will give you the mouthfeel you're looking for! As for the rest of the recipe, it will have you feeling as though your taste buds flew all the way to Vietnam to gulp down this popular street food.

2
SERVINGS

Per Serving: Calories: 461; Total Fat: 33g; Total Carbohydrates: 7g; Net Carbs: 6g; Fiber: 1g; Protein: 34g; Erythritol: 1g

Macronutrients: Fat 65%; Protein 29%; Carbs 6%

5 cups beef broth or Bone Broth (page 203)

4 lemongrass stalks, tough outer leaves and bulb removed

1 small white onion, minced

2 teaspoons minced anchovies

1 tablespoon minced peeled fresh ginger

1 teaspoon garlic powder

½ cinnamon stick

½ tablespoon tamari

½ teaspoon erythritol

Red pepper flakes (optional)

8 ounces pork shoulder

1 tablespoon avocado oil

8 ounces shirataki noodles

⅓ cup fresh cilantro, coarsely chopped

Bean sprouts (optional)

Juice of ½ lime

Sugar-free hot sauce (optional)

1. Pour the beef broth into a large pot and add the lemongrass, onion, anchovies, ginger, garlic, cinnamon stick, tamari, erythritol, and red pepper flakes to taste (if using). Bring to a boil over medium-high heat, then cover, reduce the heat to low, and let simmer for about 1 hour.

2. When you have about 15 minutes left for your pho broth, in a sauté pan over medium-high heat, sear the pork in the avocado oil for 4 to 5 minutes per side. Remove the pork from the pan and slice thinly.

3. Divide the shirataki noodles between two soup bowls.

4. Strain the pho broth and discard the solids. Divide the broth between the bowls, then add some of the pork slices, cilantro, and bean sprouts (if using) to each bowl. Garnish with lime juice and sprinkle with some hot sauce if you like your food spicy!

SWAP: *You can swap in chicken or beef for the pork if you'd prefer— pho is traditionally made with either of those meats.*

BRAND: *If you'd prefer to use fish sauce instead of anchovies, choose one that contains no sugar. I like Red Boat Fish Sauce.*

SPAGHETTI SQUASH & GROUND PORK STIR-FRY WITH KALE

PREP TIME: 10 MINUTES / COOK TIME: 1 HOUR 25 MINUTES

While I would love to give myself full credit for this recipe, I need to give my sister Daniele and her husband, Josh, a shout-out because they are the real brains behind it. I remember walking into their kitchen when they were cooking up this one-pot feast. I could smell the rosemary, garlic, onion, and oregano dancing with the sweetness of the ground pork. The addition of spaghetti squash makes it even heartier. This dish is also a great way to get antioxidant-rich kale into your diet, especially if you're not a big fan of it, much like yours truly.

BULK COOK, ONE POT

3-4
SERVINGS

Per Serving: Calories: 355; Total Fat: 23g; Total Carbohydrates: 14g; Net Carbs: 8g; Fiber: 6g; Protein: 23g

Macronutrients: Fat 60%; Protein 25%; Carbs 15%

1 medium spaghetti squash, halved lengthwise and seeded

2 tablespoons avocado or macadamia nut oil, divided

1 pound ground free-range pork

Salt

Freshly ground black pepper

1 bunch kale, stems removed, leaves chopped (2 to 3 cups)

1 teaspoon garlic powder

1 teaspoon onion powder

1 teaspoon dried parsley

½ teaspoon dry mustard powder

½ teaspoon dried rosemary

½ teaspoon dried oregano

1. Preheat the oven to 400°F. Line a baking sheet with aluminum foil.

2. Brush the cut side of the spaghetti squash with 1 tablespoon of the oil. Place it cut side down on the baking sheet and roast for 45 minutes to 1 hour, or until tender when pierced with a fork. Remove from the oven and let sit until cool enough to handle.

3. In a large skillet or a wok, heat the oil over medium-high heat. Add the ground pork and season with salt and pepper. Cook for about 5 minutes, stirring and breaking the meat up into pieces.

4. Scoop the squash flesh (the spaghetti strands) into the skillet or wok and stir to combine with the meat. Reserve the spaghetti squash shells for serving, if you'd like.

5. Add the kale, garlic and onion powders, parsley, dry mustard powder, rosemary, oregano, and salt and pepper to taste. Mix everything together until well combined and cook for 10 minutes, or until the meat is no longer pink and the kale is wilted.

6. To serve, scoop the pork mixture into the reserved spaghetti squash shells or simply serve up in bowls or on plates!

TIP: *Cooking spaghetti squash in bulk is a great idea since it will keep in the refrigerator for up to 5 days.*

SWAP: *You can use ground beef, lamb, or wild boar for this recipe instead of the ground pork.*

BEEF BURGERS WITH BACON

PREP TIME: 10 MINUTES / COOK TIME: 30 MINUTES

Now that you know sugar-free, free-range bacon is a power food in the keto world, feel free to include it as often as you can—like in the meat of your burger. Doing this is never a mis-steak!

2-4
SERVINGS

Per Serving: Calories: 413;
Total Fat: 33g; Total
Carbohydrates: 3g; Net Carbs:
2g; Fiber: 1g; Protein: 26g

Macronutrients: Fat 72%;
Protein 25%; Carbs 3%

2 slices sugar-free beef or pork bacon

1 pound ground beef

½ teaspoon onion powder

½ teaspoon garlic powder

½ teaspoon nutmeg

½ teaspoon dried sage

¼ teaspoon dried oregano or marjoram

Salt

Freshly ground black pepper

4 to 8 thick cabbage leaves, or more for crunch

Sliced grass-fed/-finished cheese, for serving (optional)

Sliced tomato and raw or grilled onion slices, for serving (optional)

2 to 4 fried eggs, for serving (optional)

Chipotle-lime or plain mayonnaise (optional)

1. In a shallow sauté pan over medium-high heat, fry up the bacon to your desired doneness, flipping once, 5 to 8 minutes. (There is no need to add extra cooking fat, as the bacon is fatty enough, but if you haven't gotten your allotment of fat yet for the day, feel free to add some butter or oil to the pan.)

2. Remove the bacon from the pan, let cool, then cut into small pieces. Do not wipe out the pan.

3. In a mixing bowl, combine the ground beef with the bacon pieces, onion and garlic powders, nutmeg, sage, and oregano. Season with salt and pepper. With clean hands, mix together until well combined, then form into burger patties.

4. Place the same skillet that you used for the bacon over medium-high heat, add the burgers, and cook to your desired doneness, 3 to 4 minutes per side for medium-rare.

5. Place a thick piece of cabbage or two on each serving plate, then top with a burger. If you'd like, top with cheese, then add some tomato and onion slices. If you want, you can also top your burger with a fried egg.

6. Slather the remaining cabbage leaves with mayonnaise (if using), then sandwich everything together and enjoy!

TIP: *When cleaning your pan after creating this recipe, it's best to scrape all the fat and grease left in the pan into the trash. If you pour it down your sink or garbage disposal, you might clog your drain.*

SLOW-COOKED SHREDDED BEEF

PREP TIME: 10 MINUTES / COOK TIME: 6 HOURS

While I love speedy recipes, once in a while slow and steady wins the race. Patience will pay off with this succulent and rich beef recipe. Since it takes a while for the beef to tenderize, you can make a few different side dishes to complement the main event while you wait!

**BULK COOK,
ONE POT**

4–5
SERVINGS

Per Serving: Calories: 480;
Total Fat: 36g; Total
Carbohydrates: 5g; Net Carbs:
4g; Fiber: 1g; Protein: 34g

Macronutrients: Fat 68%;
Protein 28%; Carbs 4%

TIP: *If you don't have
an oven-safe Dutch
oven or pot, then you
can make this dish
on the stovetop; just
turn the heat to low
and simmer for about
6 hours there. If you use
an Instant Pot, your
cooking time will be
reduced substantially.*

SWAP: *You can make
this recipe using a pork
roast, as well.*

2 pounds beef chuck roast

2 teaspoons salt

1 teaspoon freshly ground black pepper

1 teaspoon garlic powder

1 teaspoon onion powder

1 teaspoon paprika

1 teaspoon oregano

3 tablespoons avocado oil or macadamia nut oil

1 onion, quartered

2 garlic cloves, peeled

1½ cups sugar-free beef broth or Bone Broth (page 203)

1. Preheat the oven to 275°F.

2. Put the beef chuck roast in a large mixing bowl and add the salt, pepper, garlic and onion powders, paprika, and oregano. Massage with your hands to coat the roast completely with the seasonings.

3. In an oven-safe Dutch oven, heat the oil over medium-high heat. Add the roast and brown on all sides, 3 to 5 minutes per side.

4. Add the onion, garlic, and broth, then cover the pot, transfer to the oven, and cook for about 6 hours, or until fork-tender.

5. Remove the roast from the pot, transfer to a cutting board, and use two forks to shred the meat. At this point, you can transfer the meat back to the pot to absorb more of the flavors from the broth, and serve from there.

BEEF STROGANOFF

PREP TIME: 10 MINUTES / COOK TIME: 20 TO 25 MINUTES

Until I tried making my own variation of beef Stroganoff, I always thought the pairing of dairy products with beef was weird, despite both ingredients coming from the same source. I promise, though, that you won't want to miss out on this creamy yet bold flavor combination, originally invented by a French chef during a Russian cooking competition in 1891.

2 pounds beef tenderloin or sirloin steak, sliced into strips

Salt

Freshly ground black pepper

4 tablespoons butter, ghee, or butter-flavored coconut oil, divided

1 white onion, diced

2 cups button mushrooms, sliced

2 garlic cloves, minced

¼ cup almond flour, or 2 tablespoons coconut flour plus 2 tablespoons arrowroot flour

3 cups Bone Broth (page 203)

2 teaspoons tamari

¼ teaspoon freshly squeezed lemon juice

¼ teaspoon erythritol

Splash sugar-free hot sauce

1 teaspoon Dijon mustard

1 teaspoon paprika

¼ cup sugar-free plain Greek or coconut yogurt

3 cups shirataki noodles, well drained, or other cooked vegetable noodles

Chopped fresh parsley, for garnish (optional)

BULK COOK, ONE POT

8
SERVINGS

Per Serving: Calories: 400; Total Fat: 27g; Total Carbohydrates: 7g; Net Carbs: 6g; Fiber: 1g; Protein: 36g

Macronutrients: Fat 60%; Protein 35%; Carbs 5%

1. Season the beef with salt and pepper.

2. Melt 2 tablespoons of butter in a large, shallow skillet over medium-high heat. Add the beef and brown on both sides, 2 to 4 minutes total. Remove the beef from the pan and set aside on a plate.

BEEF STROGANOFF *continues*

SWAP: *While beef Stroganoff is a very traditional recipe, don't be scared to mix it up and use another cut of meat if you're not feeling the beef. Chicken tenderloin is another option, or you can even use whitefish like halibut or swordfish.*

3. In the same skillet, melt the remaining 2 tablespoons of butter, then add the onion, mushrooms, and garlic. Cook the vegetables for 4 minutes, then add the almond flour and stir to evenly combine.

4. Stir in the broth, reduce the heat to low, and continue stirring until thickened, 3 to 5 minutes.

5. Add the tamari, lemon juice, erythritol, hot sauce, mustard, paprika, and yogurt. Stir everything together again, then add the beef and let simmer for 5 to 8 minutes, or until the beef is browned and juicy.

6. Either add the shirataki noodles to the skillet and toss to combine with the sauce, or divide the noodles among bowls and pour the sauce over them. Top with parsley, if desired.

PORK CHOPS SMOTHERED IN CARAMELIZED ONIONS & LEEKS

PREP TIME: 5 TO 10 MINUTES / COOK TIME: 20 MINUTES

You may find your taste buds squealing with delight over this recipe, and you'll want to hog it all to yourself. This dish is so light yet flavorful. It is both savory and a bit sweet. Pork, which is rich in thiamine (vitamin B1), is a sweet white meat, so when topped with caramelized onion and leeks, the whole thing explodes with deep flavors. It's time you pig out on this insanely easy-to-make palate pleaser! It'll be even better served with Cauliflower "Potato" Salad (page 95), Cauliflower Mac & Cheese (page 113), or some roasted Brussels sprouts and fennel.

2 bone-in free-range pork chops

1 teaspoon salt

1 teaspoon freshly ground black pepper

2 tablespoons avocado oil, divided

1 tablespoon butter or butter-flavored coconut oil

1 red onion, thinly sliced

1 leek, white and light green parts thinly sliced

1. Season the pork chops on both sides with the salt and pepper.

2. Heat 1 tablespoon of avocado oil in a shallow skillet over medium-high heat. Add the butter to melt.

3. Lay the pork chops in the pan and cook until golden brown, about 3 minutes, then flip and cook on the other side for 3 to 5 minutes, until no longer pink on the inside and golden brown on the outside.

4. In another skillet, heat the remaining tablespoon of avocado oil over medium-high heat. Add the onion and leek and cook until translucent, 5 to 8 minutes.

5. Transfer the pork chops to plates and top with the sautéed onion and leek.

BULK COOK, SUPER QUICK

2
SERVINGS

Per Serving: Calories: 480; Total Fat: 32g; Total Carbohydrates: 12g; Net Carbs: 9g; Fiber: 3g; Protein: 36g

Macronutrients: Fat 60%; Protein 30%; Carbs 10%

TIP: *It's smart (and even more delicious) to buy bone-in pork chops because they typically come from a fattier, more flavorful part of the pig.*

SWAP: *To reduce the bite, swap fennel or another leek for the red onion.*

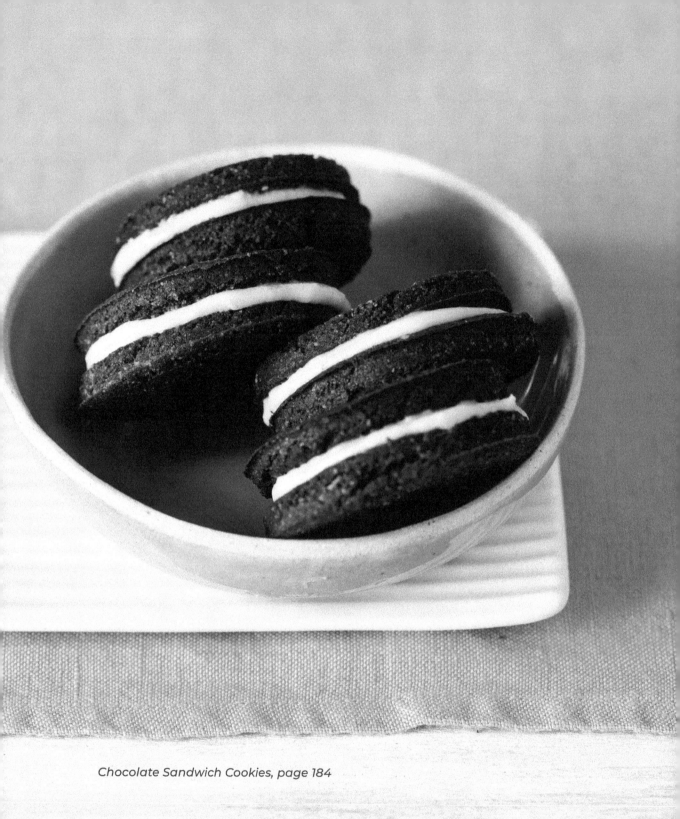

Chocolate Sandwich Cookies, page 184

Chapter 9

Desserts

Birthday parties, holidays, staff meetings, kids' school events, a random Tuesday evening—life is full of celebrations that call for sweet treats! These recipes are here to cater to those special events.

Dairy-Free White Chocolate Bark 180

Simple Ice Cream with 8 Flavor Customizations 181

Avocado Brownies 183

Chocolate Sandwich Cookies 184

Sweet Egg Salad 186

Air-Fried Vanilla and Chocolate Layer Cake 188

Snickerdoodle Pudding 190

Churros 191

Cake or Cookie Dough Balls 193

DAIRY-FREE WHITE CHOCOLATE BARK

PREP TIME: 15 MINUTES (PLUS 2 HOURS OF FREEZING TIME)

I have to confess that I am not a chocolate lover. But white chocolate is a whole other story. I was a huge fan of white chocolate bars when I was a kid, so I had to try to re-create my favorite one to exclude the sugar, flour, and hydrogenated oils, yet include lauric acid, a saturated fat used for treating viral infections such as the flu.

BULK COOK

MAKES
12
PIECES OF BARK

Per Serving (1 ounce,
so maybe 8 servings):
Calories: 176; Total Fat: 16g;
Total Carbohydrates: 5g;
Net Carbs: 2g; Fiber: 3g;
Protein: 3g; Erythritol: 12g

Macronutrients: Fat 82%;
Protein 11%; Carbs 7%

Nonstick cooking spray
6 ounces coconut butter
1 ounce coconut oil
¼ cup keto-approved protein powder
¼ cup powdered erythritol
2 tablespoons unsweetened coconut milk
1 teaspoon vanilla extract
1 teaspoon cookie/cake flavor extract (or more vanilla extract)
2 tablespoons sugar-free chocolate chips

1. Coat a small baking dish with nonstick spray.

2. In a blender, combine the coconut butter, coconut oil, protein powder, erythritol, coconut milk, and vanilla and cookie/cake extracts. Blend until completely smooth.

3. Pour the contents of the blender evenly into the prepared baking dish. Sprinkle with the chocolate chips and freeze for at least 2 hours before cutting or breaking into pieces and digging in.

SWAP: *You can easily make this recipe with dairy products. Instead of coconut butter, use regular butter; instead of coconut milk, use whole cow's milk and omit the coconut oil.*

SIMPLE ICE CREAM WITH 8 FLAVOR CUSTOMIZATIONS

PREP TIME: 5 MINUTES (PLUS 24 HOURS PLUS 30 MINUTES OF FREEZING TIME)

I've heard people say that ice cream solves everything. Unfortunately, for keto folks, that's just not the case. Enter this recipe! With its many variations, it's here to solve the ice cream problem, because it puts you in complete control of what goes into the creamy mix!

FOR ICE CREAM BASE

1 (13.5-ounce) can full-fat coconut milk or 1 pint heavy (whipping) cream

⅓ cup granulated or powdered erythritol

¼ cup keto-approved vanilla protein powder

¼ cup water

1 teaspoon vanilla extract

3-4
SERVINGS

Per Serving: Calories: 248; Total Fat: 24g; Total Carbohydrates: 2g; Net Carbs: 2g; Fiber: 0g; Protein: 6g; Erythritol: 18g

Macronutrients: Fat 87%; Protein 10%; Carbs 3%

1. Freeze the bowl of an ice cream maker for at least 24 hours prior to making the ice cream.

2. Place the coconut milk or cream in a mixing bowl and stir in the erythritol, protein powder of choice (depending on which flavor you're making), water, and vanilla extract. To make a specific flavor, either add the appropriate ingredients now, or add them halfway through the ice cream making process in the next step.

3. Transfer the milk mixture to the frozen bowl and situate in the ice cream maker. Place the ice cream blade into the bowl and cover with the plastic top. Turn the ice cream maker on and watch as the magic happens. It will take 25 to 30 minutes to reach the thick, creamy consistency you're looking for.

4. Spoon the ice cream into bowls. Garnish with the optional toppings for whichever flavor you made.

SIMPLE ICE CREAM WITH
8 FLAVOR CUSTOMIZATIONS *continues*

TIP: *If you don't have an ice cream maker, use a blender. The consistency will be a bit different, though.*

FOR VANILLA

1 teaspoon vanilla extract

Vanilla bean, for topping (optional)

FOR CHOCOLATE CHIP

½ cup sugar-free chocolate chips

FOR MINT CHIP

35 drops peppermint stevia extract

1 square unsweetened dark or peppermint dark chocolate

FOR CHOCOLATE

¼ cup keto-approved chocolate protein powder or ¼ cup cocoa powder plus 20 drops chocolate stevia extract (instead of vanilla protein powder)

FOR STRAWBERRY

¼ cup keto-approved strawberry protein powder or 1 teaspoon strawberry flavor extract plus ½ cup sliced strawberries (instead of vanilla protein powder)

FOR PISTACHIO

½ cup shelled pistachios

½ teaspoon almond extract

FOR BUTTER PECAN

½ cup pecans

1 tablespoon butter, butter-flavored coconut oil, or butter flavor extract

1 teaspoon erythritol "brown sugar"

FOR COCONUT

1 tablespoon coconut extract

¼ cup puréed coconut meat

2 tablespoons coconut flakes, for topping (optional)

AVOCADO BROWNIES

PREP TIME: 5 TO 10 MINUTES / COOK TIME: 25 MINUTES

Even though I'm not into straight-up chocolate, these brownies are totally my thing thanks to the monounsaturated-fat-laden avocado. The avocado creates the most luscious, creamy consistency that'll make you think you're eating fudge. And guess what? These brownies are roughly 10 million times healthier than those made from store-bought mixes. Fudge, these are good!

Nonstick cooking spray or 1 tablespoon coconut oil

1 avocado, halved, pitted, and peeled

2 tablespoons keto-approved vanilla protein powder

2 tablespoons keto-approved chocolate protein powder

¼ cup unsweetened cocoa powder

¼ cup erythritol

1 egg

1½ teaspoons vanilla extract

3 tablespoons unsweetened coconut milk

Powdered erythritol or Simple Ice Cream (page 181), for serving

1. Preheat the oven to 350°F. Coat a baking dish with nonstick spray or coconut oil.

2. In a blender, combine the avocado, protein powders, cocoa, erythritol, egg, vanilla extract, and coconut milk and purée until smooth.

3. Pour the avocado brownie batter evenly into the prepared baking dish and bake for 20 to 25 minutes, or until a toothpick inserted in the center comes out clean.

4. Let the brownies cool for at least 10 minutes, then slice into squares and serve with a sprinkle of powdered erythritol or the ice cream flavor of your choice.

BULK COOK

MAKES
12-14
BROWNIES

Per Serving: Calories: 61; Total Fat: 5g; Total Carbohydrates: 2g; Net Carbs: 1g; Fiber: 2g; Protein: 2g; Erythritol: 4g

Macronutrients: Fat 74%; Protein 13%; Carbs 13%

TIP: *These brownies are amazing paired with vanilla ice cream.*

SWAP: *If you want to make blondies, omit the cocoa and use only vanilla protein powder. They may look more like "gree-nies" because of the avocado, but don't be scared off—this ver-sion is delicious, too.*

CHOCOLATE SANDWICH COOKIES

PREP TIME: 20 MINUTES / COOK TIME: 15 MINUTES

Many people love Oreos, so I made my own version of the blissful sandwich cookie, and it's teeming with health benefits! In the past, you may have berated yourself for eating a whole sleeve of Oreos in one sitting, but with these cookies, you can feel good about chowing down!

BULK COOK

MAKES
7
SANDWICH COOKIES

Per Serving (1 sandwich cookie): Calories: 368; Total Fat: 24g; Total Carbohydrates: 28g; Net Carbs: 16g; Fiber: 12g; Protein: 10g

Macronutrients: Fat 60%; Protein 12%; Carbs 28%

FOR THE COOKIES
¼ cup coconut flour
¼ cup unsweetened cocoa powder
¼ cup water
2 tablespoons tapioca flour
2 tablespoons glucomannan powder or xanthan gum
4 tablespoons coconut butter
1 tablespoon unsweetened coconut milk
1 egg
1 teaspoon vanilla extract
2 tablespoons xylitol-sweetened honey
1 tablespoon erythritol

FOR THE CREAM FILLING
3 tablespoons coconut butter, melted
1 tablespoon keto-approved vanilla protein powder
2 tablespoons water
½ teaspoon vanilla extract
1 tablespoon xylitol-sweetened honey

MAKE THE COOKIES

1. Preheat the oven to 350°F. Line a baking sheet with parchment paper.

2. In a mixing bowl, combine the coconut flour, cocoa powder, water, tapioca flour, glucomannan powder, coconut butter, coconut milk, egg, vanilla extract, honey, and erythritol and mix together well.

3. Transfer the cookie dough to the prepared baking sheet and use a rolling pin to roll out ⅛ inch thick.

4. Bake in the oven for about 15 minutes, or until soft but no longer sticky.

MAKE THE CREAM FILLING AND ASSEMBLE

1. While the cookies are baking, in a mixing bowl, combine the coconut butter, protein powder, water, vanilla extract, and honey and whisk until smooth.

2. Remove the baked cookie dough from the oven and let cool for at least 5 minutes. Then use a round cookie cutter to cut out 12 or 14 cookies.

3. Let the cut-out cookies continue to cool for 15 to 20 minutes (you can put in the refrigerator to cool faster).

4. Spread the cream filling on one side of half of the cookies, then sandwich together with the remaining cookies and serve.

TIP: *If you cut out your cookies prior to baking, you can use the remaining cookie dough to make even more sandwich cookies by repeating steps 3 and 4.*

SWAP: *If you want to make "golden" sandwich cookies, omit the cocoa powder in the cookie dough recipe.*

BRAND: *Nature's Hollow is the brand of xylitol-sweetened honey I use for this recipe.*

SWEET EGG SALAD

PREP TIME: 5 MINUTES / COOK TIME: 10 MINUTES

Who says you can't swap out savory ingredients in a typical egg salad recipe for sweet ones? The results of this eggsperiment were so eggsciting that I had to include this recipe in this book. I would eggsplain the flavors and textures in greater detail, but they're really something you need to eggsplore for yourself! Does this recipe leave your brain a bit scrambled? Well, let me assure you that it's no yolk and, if I do say so myself, it's quite eggscellent! (Seriously, though, it's weird, but it's good.)

SUPER QUICK

4
SERVINGS

Per Serving: Calories: 154; Total Fat: 10g; Total Carbohydrates: 5g; Net Carbs: 3g; Fiber: 2g; Protein: 11g; Erythritol: 4.5g

Macronutrients: Fat 58%; Protein 29%; Carbs 13%

6 eggs

1 scoop keto-approved vanilla protein powder

1½ tablespoons powdered erythritol

1 teaspoon vanilla extract

1 tablespoon unsweetened coconut milk (optional)

½ cup sugar-free chocolate chips

Sugar-free syrup and melted butter-flavored coconut oil, for serving (optional)

1. Fill a large bowl with ice and water.

2. Place the eggs in a large pot filled with water and bring to a boil. Cook for 10 to 12 minutes.

3. Using a slotted spoon, carefully transfer the eggs to the ice bath to cool for 3 minutes, then peel the eggs and put in a large mixing bowl.

4. Add the protein powder, erythritol, vanilla extract, and coconut milk (if using) to the bowl and mash everything together.

5. Add the chocolate chips and mix everything together again.

6. Serve the egg salad drizzled, if you'd like, with syrup or the melted coconut oil.

TIP: *If you do not have sugar-free chocolate chips on hand, crush a sugar-free chocolate bar into pieces to use instead.*

SWAP: *You can opt for regular cow's milk and butter in this recipe. If you would prefer an even faster recipe, scramble the eggs instead of hard-boiling them, then add all the other ingredients to the scramble.*

BRAND: *Hershey's sells sugar-free chocolate chips, but they contain milk. If you need a vegan variety, look for Lily's brand.*

AIR-FRIED VANILLA AND CHOCOLATE LAYER CAKE

PREP TIME: 15 MINUTES / COOK TIME: 1 HOUR

Who would have thought you could have your cake and keto, too? Well, you certainly can with this rendition of sponge cake that is just oh-so sweet. And since I know many people love chocolate, I made a chocolate layer of this sweet treat to satisfy those cravings, too!

8
SERVINGS

Per Serving: Calories: 620; Total Fat: 52g; Total Carbohydrates: 22g; Net Carbs: 10g; Fiber: 12g; Protein: 16g; Erythritol: 24g

Macronutrients: Fat 75%; Protein 11%; Carbs 14%

FOR THE CAKE LAYERS
Nonstick cooking spray

1 cup coconut flour, divided

¼ cup keto-approved vanilla protein powder

1 cup melted butter-flavored coconut oil, divided

1 cup erythritol, divided

1 teaspoon baking soda, divided

10 eggs, divided

¼ cup coconut milk, divided

24 drops vanilla-flavored liquid stevia, divided

2 tablespoons unsweetened cocoa powder

FOR THE FROSTING
½ cup melted butter-flavored coconut oil

¼ cup unsweetened cocoa powder

12 to 24 drops vanilla-flavored liquid stevia

2 tablespoons sugar-free coconut yogurt (optional but recommended)

MAKE THE CAKE LAYERS

1. Spray a small round cake pan (small enough to fit in an air fryer) with nonstick spray.

2. In a blender, combine ½ cup of coconut flour, the vanilla protein powder, ½ cup of coconut oil, ½ cup of erythritol, ½ teaspoon of baking soda, 5 eggs, 2 tablespoons of coconut milk, and 12 drops of liquid stevia and purée until smooth.

3. Pour the vanilla cake batter into the prepared pan, place in the air fryer and air-fry at 400°F for 12 to 15 minutes, or until nicely browned and a spatula can be inserted around the edge without the cake sticking to it.

4. Remove the vanilla layer from the air fryer. Invert onto a plate, then return to the cake pan and put back in the air fryer to cook on the other side. Reduce the temperature to 370°F and bake for another 15 minutes, or until nicely browned and a toothpick inserted in the center comes out clean. Remove from the air fryer and let cool for 20 to 30 minutes.

5. Using the remaining cake ingredients, repeat steps 1 through 3 to make the chocolate layer, but use the chocolate protein powder instead of vanilla and add the cocoa powder. Let cool for 20 to 30 minutes when done baking.

MAKE THE FROSTING AND ASSEMBLE THE CAKE

1. In a mixing bowl, combine the oil with the cocoa powder, liquid stevia, and coconut yogurt (if using), then mix until it forms a frosting-like consistency.

2. Arrange the cake layers on top of one another in whatever order you prefer, then use a butter knife to spread the frosting all over the cake. (If you don't let the cake layers cool long enough, the icing will melt right off, so it's a *very* good idea to let them cool as long as possible.)

3. Slice the cake into pieces, divvy up on plates, grab a fork (if you're classy, unlike me), and dive in!

TIP: *To tell if a cake layer is done, grab a toothpick and stick it in the center of the cake. If you pull it out and there is batter stuck to it, then it still needs more time. If the toothpick is clean, then the cake is ready to be removed from the oven.*

SWAP: *If you don't have an air fryer, you can make this recipe in the oven; just preheat the oven first. Baking in the oven will take 25 minutes less since you can cook both layers of cake at the same time.*

SNICKERDOODLE PUDDING

PREP TIME: 3 MINUTES

When I think of pudding, I am reminded of those individual puddings that were all the rage in grade school cafeterias. Now that I've got you craving that creamy treat, let me introduce you to a new and improved pudding snack, without the sugar, modified corn starch, and omega-6-laden vegetable oil. Aside from the healthy monounsaturated fats from the avocado that will keep you feeling satisfied, the greatest part about this recipe is that you can customize the flavor however you'd like. This snickerdoodle flavor will have you licking your pudding bowl clean, but you can alter it as you wish.

BULK COOK, SUPER QUICK

1
SERVING

Per Serving: Calories: 268; Total Fat: 16g; Total Carbohydrates: 7g; Net Carbs: 6g; Fiber: 5g; Protein: 20g; Syrup Carbs: 60g (syrup fiber: 56g)

Macronutrients: Fat 54%; Protein 30%; Carbs 16%

¼ cup keto-approved vanilla protein powder

½ avocado, pitted and peeled

¼ cup sugar-free cinnamon maple syrup

1 teaspoon vanilla extract

½ tablespoon ground cinnamon

1 tablespoon coconut or almond flour (optional)

1 tablespoon erythritol (optional)

1 tablespoon collagen to end of ingredients list

1. In a blender or food processor, combine the protein powder, avocado, maple syrup, vanilla, cinnamon, flour, collagen, and erythritol (if using), and blend until smooth.

2. Serve the pudding in a bowl and enjoy as a light snack on the days you feel ravenous!

TIP: *Make this recipe in bulk, pour it into ice cube trays, then freeze. You can eat the cubes as tasty snacks on their own or put them in a blender and make a frothy smoothie or ice cream shake.*

SWAP: *You can use pumpkin instead of avocado in this recipe. However, if you swap pumpkin in, add 1 tablespoon of melted coconut oil or butter to make up for the lack of fat. To make it similar to the consistency of avocado, you may need to add xanthan gum or guar gum, both thickening agents.*

CHURROS

PREP TIME: 5 TO 10 MINUTES / COOK TIME: 15 TO 40 MINUTES

I remember quite vividly the one and only time I ever had a bite of a churro. I was at an amusement park, and after taking that bite, my thinking got fuzzy and my eyesight got blurry. I thought I was dying and going to heaven because of the cinnamon-sugar bliss. I didn't have a churro again until I made this keto-approved variation that is actually better than the bite of bliss I had so long ago. The best part is, it's far more nutritious!

½ cup keto-approved vanilla protein powder

½ cup coconut flour

½ cup unsweetened coconut milk

¾ cup water

2 eggs

2 tablespoons erythritol

¼ cup coconut oil, divided

1 tablespoon ground cinnamon

1 tablespoon baking soda

Powdered erythritol and sugar-free cinnamon maple syrup, for serving (optional)

MAKES
6
CHURROS

Per Serving: Calories: 319; Total Fat: 19g; Total Carbohydrates: 15g; Net Carbs: 6g; Fiber: 9g; Protein: 22g; Erythritol: 4g

Macronutrients: Fat 54%; Protein 27%; Carbs 19%

1. In a large mixing bowl, combine the protein powder, coconut flour, coconut milk, water, eggs, erythritol, 2 tablespoons of coconut oil, cinnamon, and baking soda. Mix until smooth. (You can also do this in a food processor or blender.)

2. Get a gallon-size zip-top bag, snip one corner of it with scissors, and fill with the churro batter.

3. Heat the remaining 2 tablespoons of coconut oil in a shallow skillet over medium-high heat. Pipe two or three strips of the churro batter into the skillet and cook for about 3 minutes per side, or until they have a nice crisp crust. (Be careful: The coconut oil will get very hot and could "pop" in your face and splash you.)

CHURROS *continues*

SWAP: *Are you more of a chocolate lover than a vanilla lover? Then make these churros chocolate by swapping in chocolate protein powder for vanilla and adding a tablespoon or two of cocoa powder.*

4. As the churros finish cooking, transfer them to a paper towel–lined plate to drain and cool. Continue cooking churros with the remaining batter.

5. If you'd like, serve the churros sprinkled with powdered erythritol and with maple syrup for dipping.

TIP: *While traditional churros have distinct ridges in them, the plastic bag used in this recipe leaves them smooth. If you have a piping bag with the specific nozzle to achieve the ridges, you can use that instead.*

CAKE OR COOKIE DOUGH BALLS

PREP TIME: 10 MINUTES (PLUS 1 HOUR FREEZING TIME)

This recipe makes me nostalgic because it was one of the first ever video recipes I posted on my blog, GiGi Eats Celebrities. I don't actually recommend you watch that video, though, because the production quality is horrific. That said, these cake or cookie dough balls are, as I used to say at the end of each video, scrumptious.

2 scoops keto-approved protein powder

2 tablespoons coconut flour

2 teaspoons erythritol

1 tablespoon coconut oil

4 drops cake batter flavor extract or 1½ teaspoons vanilla extract

¼ cup water or unsweetened nondairy milk of choice

2 teaspoons sugar-free chocolate chips (optional)

2 teaspoons freeze-dried strawberries (optional)

2 teaspoons nuts of your choice (optional)

2 teaspoons cocoa powder (optional)

1. In a large mixing bowl, combine the protein powder, coconut flour, erythritol, coconut oil, cake batter extract, water or milk, and, if using, the chocolate chips, strawberries, nuts, and cocoa powder. Mix until well combined and everything is evenly distributed.

2. Roll the batter into 10 to 12 balls and put on a plate. Freeze the balls for about 1 hour, if you'd like.

3. The dough balls can be enjoyed at room temperature, or you can freeze them for about 1 hour before serving. They're delicious regardless!

TIP: *I'm a big fan of making this recipe in bulk and storing it in the freezer. The dough balls keep for a long time and make the perfect post-dinner sweet treat.*

BULK COOK, SUPER QUICK

2
SERVINGS

Per Serving: Calories: 191; Total Fat: 11g; Total Carbohydrates: 11g; Net Carbs: 5g; Fiber: 6g; Protein: 12g; Erythritol: 4g

Macronutrients: Fat 52%; Protein 25%; Carbs 23%

SWAP: *To use almond flour instead of coconut flour in this recipe, just use less liquid.*

BRAND: *One on One Flavors has great flavor extracts, such as Honey Oats, Cinnamon Crunch Cereal, Peanut Butter, Coffee, and Donut.*

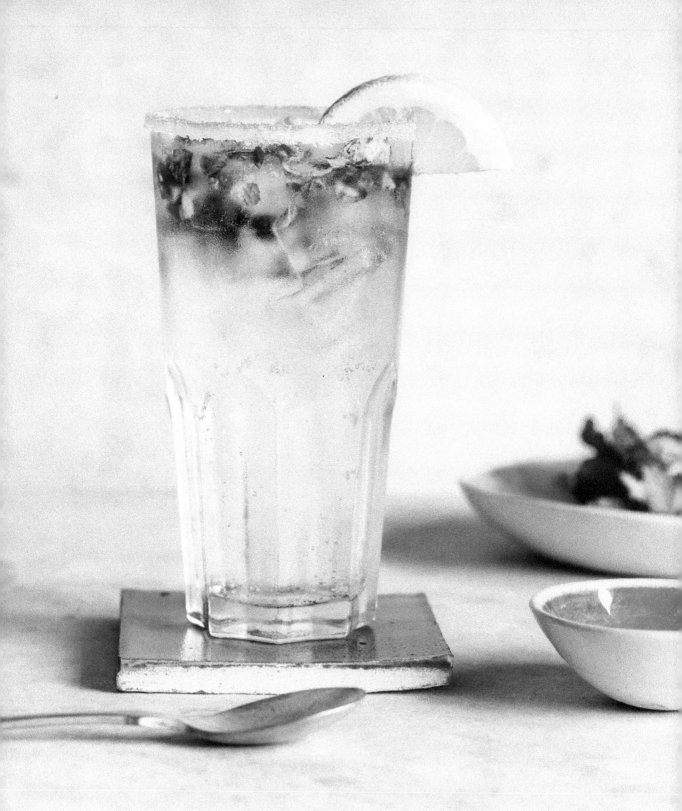

Virgin (or Not) Mojito, page 202

Chapter 10

Beverages

———

Allow me to quench your thirst. Once in a while, vivid images of Frappuccinos or the sweet alcoholic beverages you used to gulp down may start to dance in your head. I get it, which is why I created the recipes in this section. Remember some of the macronutrient ratios for these drinks are not ketogenic, but these drinks are not meant to be consumed alone.

Pumpkin Pie Smoothie **196**

Virgin (or Not) Eggnog **197**

Pumpkin Spice Latte **198**

Cauliflower Smoothie **199**

Virgin (or Not) Bloody Mary **200**

Virgin (or Not) Mojito **202**

Bone Broth **203**

Hot Cocoa/Chocolate Milk **205**

PUMPKIN PIE SMOOTHIE

PREP TIME: 5 MINUTES

I have always been fond of the holiday season. When I was a kid, I loved it because that's when the pumpkin pies would be in full bloom. Those pies did not stand a chance with me around: that crispy yet flaky cinnamon-studded buttery crust, paired with a creamy, rich, and sweet pumpkin filling. I would be lying if I said I have never polished off an entire pie in one sitting. Nowadays I polish off this pumpkin pie smoothie instead, inhaling the same delicious flavors without all that sugar and trans fat. Feel free to consume with the aid of a spoon!

SUPER QUICK

2
SERVINGS

Per Serving: Calories: 438; Total Fat: 30g; Total Carbohydrates: 28g; Net Carbs: 13g; Fiber: 13g; Protein: 14g; Erythritol Carbs: 12g

Macronutrients: Fat 62%; Protein 13%; Carbs 25%

TRIVIA: *Hemp is one of the few complete protein sources that has all the essential amino acids. On top of that, it also contains lots of essential healthy fats, such as ALA, which is an omega-3 fatty acid that your body cannot produce.*

1 cup canned pumpkin purée (not pumpkin pie mix)
¾ cup unsweetened coconut milk
2 tablespoons vanilla hemp protein
2 tablespoons erythritol
1 tablespoon coconut cream or coconut yogurt
1 teaspoon vanilla extract
1 teaspoon pumpkin pie spice, plus more for serving
Sugar-free maple syrup, for serving (optional)

1. In a blender, combine the pumpkin purée, hemp milk, hemp protein, erythritol, coconut cream, vanilla extract, and pumpkin pie spice and blend until smooth.

2. Pour into a glass and serve with an extra sprinkle of pumpkin pie spice, or you can drizzle some syrup on top.

TIP: *Coconut cream adds extra fat to this smoothie. If you've hit your fat quota for the day, omit it.*

SWAP: *You don't have to use hemp milk or hemp protein in this recipe; you can use whey, dairy milk, coconut milk, or almond milk instead.*

VIRGIN (OR NOT) EGGNOG

PREP TIME: 5 MINUTES

Prior to creating this recipe, I had never had eggnog. I was able to create this by reading ingredient labels and figuring out how I could alter the recipes that were not keto-approved. When I created this recipe, I was in utter shock that my taste testers raved about how it seduced their taste buds more than the non-keto concoction!

2 cups light coconut milk

1 cup full-fat coconut milk

1 scoop keto-approved vanilla protein powder or vanilla collagen powder

1 egg or 1 tablespoon chia seeds

8 tablespoons sugar-free maple or pancake syrup

1 teaspoon nutmeg, plus more for serving (optional)

½ teaspoon ground ginger

½ teaspoon allspice

Ground cinnamon

Rum (optional)

Sugar-free whipped cream (optional)

Olives, for garnish (optional)

1. In a blender, combine the coconut milks, protein powder (or collagen), egg (or chia seeds), syrup, nutmeg, ginger, allspice, and cinnamon to taste and blend until smooth.

2. Pour into a glass and, if you're feeling naughty, add some rum and a bit of whipped cream on top. Feel free to sprinkle on a little extra cinnamon or nutmeg, too.

TIP: *You can make your own whipped cream by whipping together full-fat coconut milk and powdered erythritol in a stand mixer.*

SWAP: *You can easily make this recipe with cow's milk instead of coconut milk.*

SUPER QUICK

4
SERVINGS

Per Serving: Calories: 347; Total Fat: 31g; Total Carbohydrates: 40g; Net Carbs: 10g; Fiber: 30g; Protein: 7g

Macronutrients: Fat 80%; Protein 8%; Carbs 12%

TRIVIA: *Rum has zero grams of sugar and zero grams of carbohydrates, so it's completely keto-approved.*

PUMPKIN SPICE LATTE

PREP TIME: 5 MINUTES / COOK TIME: 5 MINUTES

I literally can't even with this pumpkin spice latte! Call me basic if you want, but it's true. Pumpkin spice lattes have quite the reputation, including that they're full of sugar. Luckily that's not the case here since this recipe has zero sugar, so you can enjoy to your heart's content!

ONE POT, SUPER QUICK

1-2
SERVINGS

Per Serving: Calories: 254;
Total Fat: 18g;
Total Carbohydrates: 12g;
Net Carbs: 7g; Fiber: 5g;
Protein: 11g; Erythritol: 12g

Macronutrients: Fat 64%;
Protein 18%; Carbs 18%

TRIVIA: *Flax milk has the fewest calories per cup (25) of any milk. It also contains no protein but is full of omega-3 fatty acids, which prevent cancer, heart disease, and strokes.*

1 cup brewed coffee
½ cup unsweetened flax milk
1 scoop keto-approved vanilla protein powder
½ cup canned pumpkin purée (not pumpkin pie filling)
1 tablespoon coconut oil
1 tablespoon erythritol
½ teaspoon pumpkin pie spice, plus more for serving (optional)
1 tablespoon collagen powder (optional)
Cinnamon sticks, for garnish (optional)

1. In a medium saucepan, combine the coffee, flax milk, vanilla protein powder, pumpkin purée, coconut oil, erythritol, and pumpkin pie spice, and collagen powder (if using). Turn the heat to medium and warm the mixture for about 5 minutes.

2. Pour or spoon the latte into mugs and, if you'd like, dust a little extra pumpkin pie spice over the top and/ or garnish with cinnamon sticks.

TIP: *You can just as easily place all of these ingredients in a microwavable bowl and microwave on high for 3 minutes if you'd prefer not to use the stove.*

SWAP: *Instead of using canned pumpkin purée, you can use pumpkin flour/powder. Just know that the latte might not have as rich a flavor, and the consistency won't be as creamy.*

CAULIFLOWER SMOOTHIE

PREP TIME: 5 MINUTES

The person who loves cauliflower and its magical powers is going to love this creamy and sweet recipe. To the person who wants to throw a raw cauliflower at my head because she's annoyed at it being used for everything, just toss it over here, because I will gladly use it to make this recipe to convince you that cauliflower gets its praise for good reason. In all honesty, you won't even register that cauliflower is in this as you happily slurp it down.

1 scoop keto-approved vanilla protein powder

1 cup unsweetened coconut milk or almond milk

1½ cups frozen cauliflower

½ cup puréed butternut squash (optional)

2 tablespoons erythritol

2 teaspoons vanilla extract

1 tablespoon sugar-free chocolate chips or 3 squares sugar-free chocolate bar

Cake or Cookie Dough Balls, for serving (page 193; optional)

1. In a blender, combine the protein powder, coconut milk, frozen cauliflower, butternut squash (if using), erythritol, and vanilla extract and blend until the cauliflower is completely smooth.

2. Add the chocolate chips, set the blender to the lowest setting possible, and blend for another 30 seconds (you don't want the smoothie to turn completely chocolaty—unless you love chocolate, in which case, go for it).

3. Pour the smoothie into glasses and gulp down! Top with a few dough balls if you'd like.

TIP: *Add less liquid to this recipe and eat it with a spoon for more of a frozen custard feel.*

SWAP: *If you want the extra creaminess but don't care for butternut squash, use pumpkin or acorn squash.*

SUPER QUICK

2
SERVINGS

Per Serving: Calories: 392; Total Fat: 32g; Total Carbohydrates: 12g; Net Carbs: 6g; Fiber: 5g; Protein: 14g; Erythritol: 12g

Macronutrients: Fat 73%; Protein 14%; Carbs 13%

VIRGIN (OR NOT) BLOODY MARY

PREP TIME: 5 MINUTES

You know what I love about a Bloody Mary? I love that, depending on what's added to the mix, it can wind up being a whole balanced keto meal in itself. Many restaurants and bars go above and beyond, adding things like bacon and shrimp and an assortment of vegetables to the alcoholic (or not) beverage. While some might scoff at such additions, I applaud them, because when drinking alcohol, it's always smart to also eat something. Even if you don't add the alcohol, this beverage is sure to keep you quite satisfied.

SUPER QUICK

1-2
SERVINGS

Per Serving: Calories: 22; Total Fat: 0g; Total Carbohydrates: 5g; Net Carbs: 3g; Fiber: 2g; Protein: 2g

Macronutrients: Fat 0%; Protein 23%; Carbs 77%

15 ounces no-sugar-added tomato sauce

1 tablespoon plus 1¼ teaspoons freshly squeezed lemon juice

1½ tablespoons grated horseradish root

3 tablespoons tamari

½ teaspoon cayenne pepper

½ teaspoon paprika

½ teaspoon garlic powder

1¼ teaspoons erythritol

½ teaspoon sugar-free hot sauce

¼ teaspoon salt

¼ teaspoon freshly ground black pepper

2 sugar-free beef jerky sticks, for garnish (optional)

2 to 4 cooked shrimp, for garnish (optional)

2 strips cooked crisp bacon, for garnish (optional)

Lemon slices, for garnish (optional)

Vodka, for serving (optional)

1. Combine the tomato sauce, lemon juice, horseradish, tamari, cayenne, paprika, garlic powder, erythritol, hot sauce, salt, and pepper in a cocktail mixer or blender and shake/blend until the ingredients are well mixed.

2. Pour into glasses and, if desired, garnish with the beef jerky sticks, shrimp, bacon, and/or lemon slices. If you want to get tipsy, feel free to add vodka!

TIP: *If you have some leftover Bloody Mary mix and garnishes, mix them into scrambled eggs at your next meal.*

SWAP: *If you opt for food as garnish for your Bloody Mary, there are many options other than the ones here. You can add in pickled asparagus or green beans, olives, crab, or lobster. Really, this drink is a great way to clean out the fridge.*

TRIVIA: *There are some premade keto-approved Bloody Mary mixes out there, including one from The Real Dill.*

VIRGIN (OR NOT) MOJITO

PREP TIME: 5 MINUTES

The classic mojito has a lot going on. Its main ingredient, mint, has been shown to help relieve indigestion and fight bad breath. It's also healthy for women who are pregnant or breastfeeding, though in those cases, please enjoy only the virgin version. Virgin or not, this keto-approved beverage will certainly aid in revving your mojo.

SUPER QUICK

1
SERVING

Per Serving: Calories: 35;
Total Fat: 0g;
Total Carbohydrates: 8g;
Net Carbs: 6g; Fiber: 2g;
Protein: 1g; Erythritol: 24g

Macronutrients: Fat 0%;
Protein 9%; Carbs 91%

TRIVIA: *Lime juice is a natural hangover remedy. The acid in the fruit can ease head-aches and migraines that result from drink-ing too much.*

SWAP: *You can use Lemon Lime Zevia, a sugar-free, calorie-free fizzy beverage, in place of the club soda if you're looking for an even sweeter and more lime-forward cocktail.*

10 fresh mint leaves
¼ cup freshly squeezed lime juice
½ cup club soda
2 tablespoons erythritol, plus more for serving (optional)
Ice
1½ ounces light rum (optional)
1 lime wedge (optional)

1. On a cutting board, crush the mint leaves with the back of a spoon (you can do this in a muddler if you have one).

2. Put the mint in a large glass and pour in the lime juice and club soda. Add the erythritol, then use the spoon you crushed the mint with to mix the contents of the glass together.

3. Add ice to the glass, filling it almost to the top, then pour in the rum (if using).

4. Stir everything together and enjoy! If you'd like a fancier presentation, garnish with a lime wedge and dust with more erythritol.

TIP: *Smaller mint leaves will have a stronger flavor; bigger leaves will be more bitter.*

BONE BROTH

Bone broth became very popular a few years ago, with people buzzing about its health benefits. And it's true, this broth is insanely nutrient-dense, full of vitamins like A and K, minerals such as selenium, iron, zinc, and magnesium. Bone broth also contains gelatin (another name for collagen), which is beneficial for your joints! When drinking this bone broth be sure to pair it with a lot of fat in the meal that accompanies it!

3 to 5 pounds meat bones (marrow is best; use any type of meat you'd like)

¼ cup apple cider vinegar

12 cups water

4 celery stalks, coarsely chopped

3 onions, coarsely chopped

1 bunch fresh parsley, coarsely chopped

2 teaspoons salt

1. Put the meat bones in a huge pot or slow cooker (if you have one) and add the vinegar and water. Cook for about 2 hours over medium heat.

2. Add the celery and onion to the pot. You may also need to add more water at this point to keep everything submerged. Increase the heat to medium-high, bring to a boil, and cook for about 20 minutes.

3. Reduce the heat to low, cover, and simmer for 24 hours. (Do not leave the broth on the stovetop unattended; let cool and continue simmering the next day.)

4. Add the parsley to the pot in the last 5 to 10 minutes of cooking.

5. Using a slotted spoon or tongs, remove the meat bones from the broth and discard. Set a strainer over a pot and strain the broth, reserving the nutrient-rich veggies for snacking or another use.

BONE BROTH *continues*

ONE POT

12-14
SERVINGS

Per Serving: Calories: 30;
Total Fat: 0g;
Total Carbohydrates: 2g;
Net Carbs: 2g; Fiber: 0g;
Protein: 5g

Macronutrients: Fat 0%;
Protein 73%; Carbs 27%

BRAND: *You can easily purchase bone broth at any grocery store if you don't feel like making it. My favorite brands are Osso Good, Zoup!, Kettle & Fire, and Bonafide Provisions.*

6. Season the broth with salt, stir, and then divide among Mason jars or other airtight containers and store in the fridge for up to 3 to 4 days or the freezer for 12 to 14 months. Don't forget to pour yourself a glass first, though—you need a reward for waiting so long!

TIP: *If you're concerned about leaving a hot pot on the stove overnight, invest in a slow cooker.*

SWAP: *If you want a nonacidic bone broth, use beef or chicken broth instead of the apple cider vinegar.*

HOT COCOA/CHOCOLATE MILK

PREP TIME: 2 MINUTES / COOK TIME: 5 MINUTES (FOR HOT CHOCOLATE)

Have you heard the quote about chocolate essentially being salad because it comes from a plant? Well, this recipe is comprised of only the healthiest ingredients, thus you don't have to justify eating it by telling yourself you're eating a "salad." Unsweetened cocoa, the star ingredient here, is high in antioxidants that help prevent and slow damage to your cells. It may also have the power to lower your cholesterol levels and prevent memory decline. You know what? This recipe may actually be healthier than a salad!

⅓ cup full-fat coconut milk

1 cup unsweetened coconut milk

2 tablespoons unsweetened cocoa powder

2 tablespoons erythritol

2 to 5 drops chocolate-flavored liquid stevia

1 tablespoon collagen powder or "creamer" (optional)

Sugar-free marshmallow-flavored syrup, for serving (optional)

1. To make hot cocoa, in a small saucepan over medium-low heat, combine both coconut milks, the cocoa powder, erythritol, liquid stevia, and collagen powder (if using). Stir all of the ingredients together and warm for about 5 minutes, or to your desired temperature.

2. Pour the cocoa into a mug and add a little marshmallow syrup if you please.

3. To make chocolate milk, in a blender or mixing bowl, combine all the ingredients from step 1 and blend or mix until smooth.

4. Refrigerate for at least 1 hour before serving. You can add some marshmallow syrup here, too, if you'd like, but marshmallows are more of a hot chocolate kind of thing!

SWAP: *You can use full-fat cow's milk in place of the full-fat coconut milk. You can use almond, flax, or hemp milk in place of the unsweetened coconut milk.*

SUPER QUICK

1
SERVING

Per Serving: Calories: 298; Total Fat: 26g; Total Carbohydrates: 11g; Net Carbs: 6g; Fiber: 5g; Protein: 5g; Erythritol: 24g

Macronutrients: Fat 79%; Protein 6%; Carbs 15%

TIP: *If you don't want to use cocoa powder and sweeteners, add a few tablespoons of sugar-free chocolate syrup to your coconut milk, then stir and enjoy. Look for sugar-free chocolate syrup from brands like Lakanto and NuNaturals.*

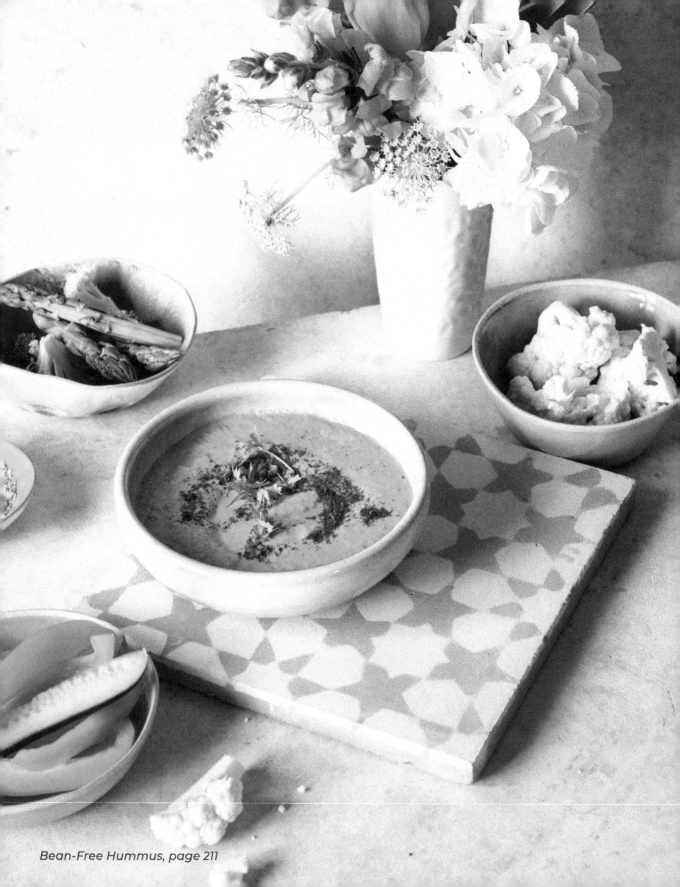

Bean-Free Hummus, page 211

Chapter 11

Sauces & Dressings

Now it's time to get saucy by making anything bland and dull into something bold and exciting!

Aioli (Fancy Mayo) **208**

Vanilla and/or Chocolate Dipping Sauce **209**

Guacamole **210**

Bean-Free Hummus **211**

Nut-Free Pesto **212**

Eggplant Dip **213**

Scampi Sauce **215**

Butternut Squash "Cheese" Sauce **216**

Yum Yum Sauce **217**

AIOLI (FANCY MAYO)

PREP TIME: 10 MINUTES

Aioli is something I will forever have a fond memory of. I knew whenever my dad made it that we were going to indulge in lobster at our next meal. I can still hear the sound of the food processor whirring away as he slowly and carefully added the olive oil to the mix, creating the deliciously creamy homemade mayonnaise. He would crack open a can of anchovies, using a few fillets to add an umami flavor to the creamy mix. Aioli is wonderful because it's not only great with lobster—you can use it for any of the recipes in this book that call for mayonnaise.

BULK COOK, SUPER QUICK

2–4
SERVINGS

Per Serving: Calories: 242;
Total Fat: 26g;
Total Carbohydrates: 1g;
Net Carbs: 1g; Fiber: 0g;
Protein: 1g

Macronutrients: Fat 96%;
Protein 2%; Carbs 2%

TIP: *This mayonnaise can be stored in an airtight container in the refrigerator for up to 1 week. Vegan version (see SWAP) can be stored for up to 2 weeks.*

1 egg yolk

1 garlic clove, minced

Salt or 3 anchovy fillets (only use one or the other)

Freshly ground black pepper

½ cup olive oil (or ¼ cup olive oil plus ¼ cup flaxseed oil for a nuttier flavor)

Juice of ¼ lemon

1 tablespoon tomato paste (optional)

Pinch paprika or red pepper flakes

1. Combine the egg yolk, garlic, salt (or anchovy fillets), and pepper to taste in a blender or food processor, cover, and start to blend on the lowest setting.

2. Carefully remove the top of the blender or open the hole on top of the food processor and, with the machine on, slowly drizzle in the oil. The mixture should start to emulsify.

3. With the machine on, add the lemon juice, tomato paste (if using), and paprika or red pepper flakes. Continue blending until smooth.

4. Use the aioli as a dipping sauce for seafood or crudités.

SWAP: *For a vegan version, use aquafaba in place of the egg yolk and add 1 tablespoon mustard. Aquafaba is the liquid that canned chickpeas are packed in. Chickpeas are not keto-approved, but the water they're soaked in is.*

VANILLA AND/OR CHOCOLATE DIPPING SAUCE

PREP TIME: 3 MINUTES

Would you find it weird if I told you that I've dunked roasted cauliflower, radishes, turnips, and jicama in these sweet sauces before? What if I told you that I've also dipped grilled chicken in them? I know, I know, but you really have to try it before you knock it! Obviously, these sauces are really meant to be drizzled over any of the Simple Ice Cream flavors (page 181) or used as a dipping sauce for the Churros (page 191), but if you think outside of the box, you can use them to sweeten up just about anything you'd like. You can even devour them with a spoon straight out of a bowl, like pudding!

1 scoop keto-approved vanilla or chocolate protein powder
½ cup unsweetened coconut milk
½ avocado, pitted and peeled
4 tablespoons xylitol-sweetened honey
1 teaspoon vanilla extract
1 to 2 tablespoons dark chocolate–flavored liquid stevia
Cocoa powder (optional)

1. In a blender or food processor, combine the vanilla or chocolate protein powder (depending on which flavor sauce you're making), the coconut milk, avocado, honey, and vanilla extract. If making chocolate sauce, add the chocolate liquid stevia and the cocoa powder (if using). Blend until smooth, about 3 minutes.

2. Serve the sauce as a dip or topping for anything you'd like, or simply eat with a spoon.

TIP: *Do not make this recipe in bulk, because you will most likely eat all of it. It's that good.*

SWAP: *Whole cow's milk can be used instead of coconut milk. You can also use almond or flax milk.*

SUPER QUICK

1
SERVING

Per Serving: Calories: 250;
Total Fat: 18g;
Total Carbohydrates: 10g;
Net Carbs: 4g; Fiber: 6g;
Protein: 12g; Xylitol Carbs: 48g

Macronutrients: Fat 65%;
Protein 19%; Carbs 16%

BRAND: *The best honey replacement I have found is made by the brand Nature's Hollow. You can find it at markets like Whole Foods or on Amazon.*

GUACAMOLE

PREP TIME: 10 MINUTES

Did you know that when you plow through a helping of guacamole, you're decreasing your risk of heart disease, lowering blood sugar levels, improving your brain health, and reviving your skin? Oh, and if you're currently pregnant, you're aiding in your baby's development thanks to the hefty amount of folate lurking within avocados. With all of those health benefits, it would be silly not to make this recipe. Pair this guac with Chicken Fajitas (page 144), use it in the Avocado "Toast" recipe (page 141), or just eat it by the spoonful.

SUPER QUICK

3-4
SERVINGS

Per Serving: Calories: 335;
Total Fat: 27g;
Total Carbohydrates: 19g;
Net Carbs: 6g; Fiber: 13g;
Protein: 4g

Macronutrients: Fat 73%;
Protein 4%; Carbs 23%

TRIVIA: *Avocado is notorious for turning brown immediately after being cut, but the way to preserve its green meaty interior for longer is by sprinkling lemon or lime juice on it, sealing in a storage container or plastic wrap, and storing in the refrigerator. It will keep for a couple of days.*

3 avocados, pitted, peeled, and chopped

½ small jalapeño pepper, seeded and minced

¼ small red onion, minced

1 small tomato or ¼ cup sun-dried tomatoes (packed in olive oil), minced

2 tablespoons chopped fresh cilantro

2 teaspoons freshly squeezed lime juice

Salt

Freshly ground black pepper

1 teaspoon garlic powder (optional)

Put the avocados in a mixing bowl and add the jalapeño, red onion, tomato, cilantro, and lime juice. Season with salt, pepper, and the garlic powder (if using) and mash everything together to your desired consistency.

TIP: *If you like your guacamole chunky, coarsely chop the onion, jalapeño pepper, and tomato, instead of mincing.*

SWAP: *I am the type of person who loves a lot of ingredients in my guacamole, so feel free to dice up bell peppers, cooked asparagus, artichoke hearts, jicama, etc., and throw them into the mix.*

BEAN-FREE HUMMUS

PREP TIME: 10 MINUTES

Hummus is a staple dip that accompanies many types of Mediterranean and Middle Eastern dishes, such as shawarma, kebabs, and gyros. Unfortunately, the keto diet isn't exactly best friends with this creamy mixture since high-carbohydrate chickpeas are the main ingredient. That's why I created a bean-free version that mimics the flavor of the real deal. Serve it with Chicken Shawarma (page 133) or as a dip for raw veggies.

2 cups chopped vegetable of choice (such as zucchini, cauliflower, or bell pepper)

½ cup tahini

¼ cup olive oil

2 tablespoons freshly squeezed lemon juice

1 tablespoon garlic powder

Salt

Freshly ground black pepper

Ground sumac or cumin, sesame seeds, and chopped fresh parsley, for serving (optional)

1. Place the chopped vegetable in a blender, add the tahini, olive oil, lemon juice, and garlic powder, and season with salt and pepper. Blend until completely smooth.

2. Serve the hummus sprinkled with sumac or cumin, sesame seeds, and chopped parsley, if you'd like.

TIP: *You can combine two or three different types of vegetable to make this hummus, but you'll need to add a bit more of the other ingredients. If you combine zucchini and cauliflower, for instance, you'll need about ¾ cup of tahini, ½ cup of olive oil, and 1½ tablespoons of garlic powder. The lemon juice in this recipe does not necessarily need to be increased, but if you love the flavor of lemons, then you certainly can.*

BULK COOK, SUPER QUICK

SERVING VARIES

Per Serving (¼ cup):
Calories: 158; Total Fat: 14g;
Total Carbohydrates: 5g;
Net Carbs: 3g; Fiber: 2g;
Protein: 3g

Macronutrients: Fat 80%;
Protein 7%; Carbs 13%

TRIVIA: *Sumac is actually made of ground-up berries from a bush that grows wild in the Mediterranean and the Middle East. This spice is a staple in Arabic cooking and is typically used instead of lemon.*

NUT-FREE PESTO

PREP TIME: 10 MINUTES / COOK TIME: 5 TO 10 MINUTES

Isn't pesto just the best-o? I certainly think it complements pretty much everything, plus pine nuts are full of healthy fats, digestion-regulating fiber, and cholesterol-lowering plant sterols. Sadly, nut allergies are on the rise, so I've created this flavorful nut-free version that uses flax meal and nutritional yeast in place of the nuts. This will still give you the nutty flavor you may crave in a pesto! Serve on top of Simply Broiled or Air-Fried Salmon (page 125) if you'd like.

BULK COOK, SUPER QUICK

SERVING VARIES

Per Serving (2 tablespoons): Calories: 96; Total Fat: 8g; Total Carbohydrates: 4g; Net Carbs: 2g; Fiber: 2g; Protein: 3g

Macronutrients: Fat 84%; Protein 6%; Carbs 10%

SWAP: *Since nuts are keto-approved, you can certainly make this pesto the traditional way with pine nuts, pecans, or Brazil nuts instead of the flax meal. Just be sure to recalculate the macros.*

15 asparagus spears, trimmed
⅓ cup fresh basil leaves, coarsely chopped
¼ cup olive oil
3 tablespoons flax meal
2 tablespoons nutritional yeast
1 tablespoon garlic powder
1 teaspoon freshly squeezed lemon juice
Salt
Freshly ground black pepper

1. Fill a pot with about ¼ inch of water and add the asparagus. Steam over medium-high heat for 5 to 10 minutes.

2. Using a slotted spoon or tongs, transfer the asparagus to a cutting board. When cool enough to handle, chop into very small pieces.

3. Put the chopped asparagus in a blender or food processor and add the basil, olive oil, flax meal, nutritional yeast, garlic powder, and lemon juice. Season with salt and pepper and blend until smooth (it's okay if larger pieces of basil remain).

TIP: *The asparagus may make the pesto a little stringy, so be sure to chop up the spears as finely as you can. If you don't like the stringiness, you can use broccoli for this recipe instead.*

EGGPLANT DIP

PREP TIME: 10 MINUTES / COOK TIME: 25 MINUTES

Eggplant is one of the most versatile vegetables, second only to cauliflower. Grilled eggplant can serve as buns for burgers or bread for cold-cut sandwiches; slices of eggplant can be used as a replacement for lasagna noodles; strands of eggplant can serve as spaghetti; and baked or broiled eggplant can be used as a vehicle for any dip you'd like to transport to your mouth. Oh, and would you look at that, eggplant can also serve as the dip! Use this one as a dip for crudités or Eggplant Chips (page 72), or slather it on chicken before baking.

2 large eggplants, halved lengthwise

½ teaspoon salt

2 tablespoons tahini

1 tablespoon Greek yogurt (optional; if using, reduce the tahini sauce by 1 tablespoon)

¼ cup olive oil

1½ garlic cloves, minced

Juice of ½ lemon

Freshly ground black pepper

Chopped fresh parsley, for garnish

4 pitted kalamata olives, for garnish (optional)

1. Preheat the oven to 400°F.

2. Season the eggplant with the salt and let sit for about 30 minutes to let the bitterness "sweat" out.

3. Wipe the eggplant off with a wet paper towel, then place cut-side up on a baking sheet. Bake in the oven for about 25 minutes, or until the eggplant flesh is fork-tender. Remove from the oven and let cool.

EGGPLANT DIP *continues*

BULK COOK

SERVING VARIES

Per Serving (1/4 cup):
Calories: 121; Total Fat: 9g;
Total Carbohydrates: 8g;
Net Carbs: 4g; Fiber: 4g;
Protein: 2g

Macronutrients: Fat 68%;
Protein 6%; Carbs 26%

TRIVIA: *Eggplant contains a flavonoid called anthocyanin, which has been found to help drop blood pressure levels. This plant pigment is also what gives the fruit (yes, fruit) its purplish color.*

4. When the eggplant is cool enough to handle, scoop out the flesh and put in a blender or food processor. Add the tahini, yogurt (if using), olive oil, garlic, lemon juice, and black pepper to taste and blend to your desired consistency. I personally like my dip a bit chunkier.

5. Serve the dip sprinkled with chopped parsley and the kalamata olives (if using).

TIP: *Don't store your eggplant in the refrigerator. Store it at room temperature and use it within a day or two.*

SWAP: *You can make this dip more Middle Eastern or Mediterranean depending on your taste preferences. If you'd like to make it more Middle Eastern, add cumin, coriander, cardamom, or sumac to the mix and sprinkle some whole sesame seeds on top. If you want to add a Mediterranean flair, add anchovies, sun-dried tomatoes, oregano, thyme, or basil.*

SCAMPI SAUCE

PREP TIME: 10 MINUTES

You might feel like a scamp for eating a recipe so rich and delicious, but you shouldn't, because scampi sauce is full of ingredients that are totally endorsed by the keto diet— even the white wine.

6 tablespoons olive or avocado oil, butter-flavored coconut oil, or melted grass-fed/-finished butter or ghee

2 tablespoons white wine

¼ cup minced shallots

4 garlic cloves, minced

2½ tablespoons chopped fresh parsley

½ tablespoon chopped fresh rosemary

½ teaspoon red pepper flakes

1 egg yolk (see Tip)

Zest of 1 lemon

Salt

Freshly ground black pepper

2 pounds cooked protein or vegetables of choice, for serving

In a bowl, whisk the oil or melted butter with the white wine, shallots, garlic, parsley, rosemary, red pepper flakes, egg yolk, lemon zest, and salt and pepper to taste. Serve the scampi sauce over whatever cooked protein or vegetables you'd like.

TIP: *You might have noticed that you'll be consuming raw egg in this sauce. Be sure to purchase free-range, pasteur-ized eggs. Only one in 30,000 eggs contains salmonella, and if you make sure to purchase your eggs from a high-quality source, you should be fine. If this makes you nervous, coat your protein or vegetables in the sauce before cooking.*

BULK COOK, SUPER QUICK

2-4
SERVINGS

Per Serving: Calories: 205; Total Fat: 21g; Total Carbohydrates: 3g; Net Carbs: 3g; Fiber: 0g; Protein: 1g

Macronutrients: Fat 92%; Protein 2%; Carbs 6%

TRIVIA: *While it should not be consumed on the regular, wine can be included on a keto-genic diet. White wine, for instance, has anywhere from 2 to 6 carbohydrates per 5 ounces. This recipe calls for only 2 tablespoons and makes 2 to 4 servings, meaning you will ingest next to no car-bohydrates at all!*

BUTTERNUT SQUASH "CHEESE" SAUCE

PREP TIME: 10 MINUTES / COOK TIME: 10 MINUTES

I used to swim in macaroni and cheese when I was younger. I would dive headfirst and then do backstrokes through that gooey cheese. Well, at least in my mind. While a cheese sauce is absolutely acceptable on the keto diet, let me introduce you to a "cheese" sauce that will make you feel as though you're doing backstrokes in the real deal. Pour this dairy-free sauce over Eggplant Chips (page 72) or vegetable noodles, or even drizzle over grilled chicken.

BULK COOK, SUPER QUICK

6

SERVINGS

Per Serving: Calories: 101; Total Fat: 5g; Total Carbohydrates: 10g; Net Carbs: 6g; Fiber: 4g; Protein: 4g

Macronutrients: Fat 45%; Protein 16%; Carbs 39%

2 cups frozen cubed butternut squash

1 tablespoon butter-flavored coconut oil

1 tablespoon tahini

2 tablespoons nutritional yeast

1 teaspoon garlic powder

½ teaspoon onion powder

½ teaspoon paprika

Salt

Freshly ground black pepper

1. In a shallow sauté pan over medium-high heat, cook the frozen butternut squash in the coconut oil until the squash is no longer frozen and the liquid in the pan has evaporated, 5 to 8 minutes.

2. Transfer the cooked squash to a blender, add the tahini, nutritional yeast, garlic and onion powders, paprika, and salt and pepper to taste. Blend until completely smooth.

TIP: *If you have leftovers of this sauce, you can freeze it in ice cube trays for future portion-sized use.*

SWAP: *Pumpkin can be used in this recipe instead of butternut squash. Warm it on the stove with coconut oil for a short period of time so it doesn't burn.*

YUM YUM SAUCE

PREP TIME: 10 MINUTES

This recipe has high expectations written all over it considering "yum" is in the name. Twice. Truth be told, it truly is quite yum yum, as it marries two staple condiments the world loves: ketchup and mayonnaise. I cannot credit myself for coming up with this combination, though, for the Japanese have been doing it for a long time. I simply re-created the sauce with keto-approved ingredients. Serve it with Pork Spring Rolls (page 164).

2 tablespoons butter or butter-flavored coconut oil, melted

1 tablespoon avocado oil mayonnaise (I use Primal Kitchen)

1 tablespoon sugar-free ketchup or tomato paste

1 teaspoon paprika

1 teaspoon garlic powder

½ teaspoon erythritol

¼ teaspoon red pepper flakes or cayenne pepper

Salt

Freshly ground black pepper

In a blender, combine the melted butter or coconut oil with the mayonnaise, ketchup or tomato paste, paprika, garlic powder, erythritol, red pepper flakes or cayenne, and salt and pepper to taste. Blend until creamy.

TIP: *If this sauce is too thick for your liking, feel free to thin it out with a little water.*

SWAP: *Avocado, olive, or algae oil can be used in place of the butter or coconut oil.*

BULK COOK, SUPER QUICK

2–3
SERVINGS

Per Serving: Calories: 169; Total Fat: 17g; Total Carbohydrates: 3g; Net Carbs: 2g; Fiber: 1g; Protein: 1g

Macronutrients: Fat 91%; Protein 2%; Carbs 7%

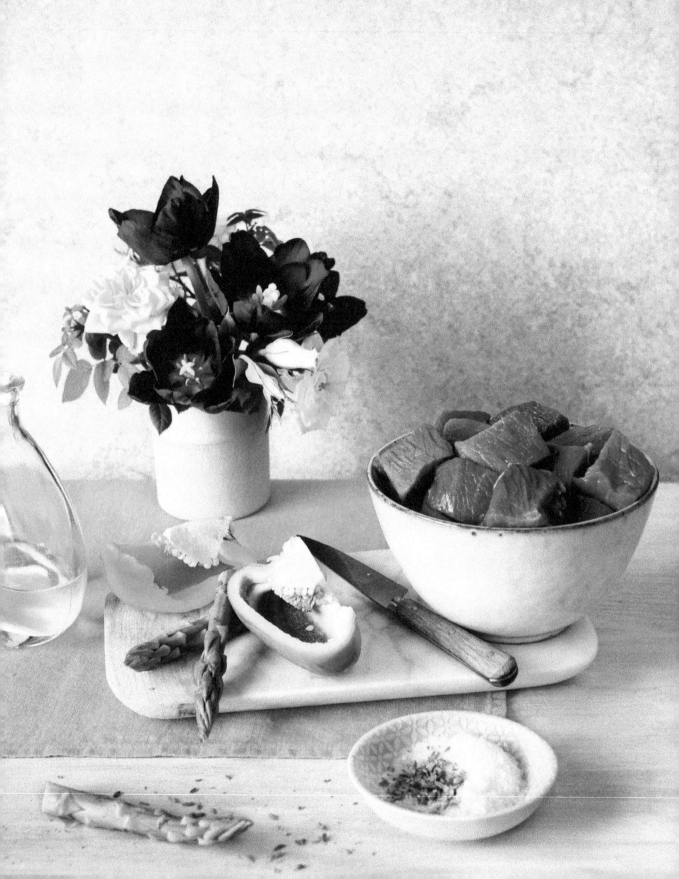

Measurement Conversions

VOLUME EQUIVALENTS (LIQUID)

US Standard	US Standard (ounces)	Metric (approximate)
2 tablespoons	1 fl. oz.	30 mL
¼ cup	2 fl. oz.	60 mL
½ cup	4 fl. oz.	120 mL
1 cup	8 fl. oz.	240 mL
1½ cups	12 fl. oz.	355 mL
2 cups or 1 pint	16 fl. oz.	475 mL
4 cups or 1 quart	32 fl. oz.	1 L
1 gallon	128 fl. oz.	4 L

OVEN TEMPERATURES

Fahrenheit (F)	Celsius (C) (approximate)
250°F	120°C
300°F	150°C
325°F	165°C
350°F	180°C
375°F	190°C
400°F	200°C
425°F	220°C
450°F	230°C

VOLUME EQUIVALENTS (DRY)

US Standard	Metric (approximate)
⅛ teaspoon	0.5 mL
¼ teaspoon	1 mL
½ teaspoon	2 mL
¾ teaspoon	4 mL
1 teaspoon	5 mL
1 tablespoon	15 mL
¼ cup	59 mL
⅓ cup	79 mL
½ cup	118 mL
⅔ cup	156 mL
¾ cup	177 mL
1 cup	235 mL
2 cups or 1 pint	475 mL
3 cups	700 mL
4 cups or 1 quart	1 L

WEIGHT EQUIVALENTS

US Standard	Metric (approximate)
½ ounce	15 g
1 ounce	30 g
2 ounces	60 g
4 ounces	115 g
8 ounces	225 g
12 ounces	340 g
16 ounces or 1 pound	455 g

References

Afaghi, A., et al. "Acute Effects of the Very Low Carbohydrate Diet on Sleep Indices." *Nutritional Neuroscience* 11, no. 4. (August 2008): 148–154. doi: 10.1179/147683008X301540.

Buyken, Anette E., et al. "Association Between Carbohydrate Quality and Inflammatory Markers: Systematic Review of Observational and Interventional Studies." *The American Journal of Clinical Nutrition* 99, no. 4. (April 2014): 813–833. doi: 10.3945/ajcn.113.074252.

Gasior, Maciej, et al. "Neuroprotective and Disease-Modifying Effects of the Ketogenic Diet." *Behavioural Pharmacology* 17, no. 5–6. (September 2006): 431–439. https://www.ncbi.nlm.nih.gov/pmc/articles/PMC2367001/

Goel, N., et al. "Sex Differences in the HPA Axis." *Comprehensive Physiology* 4, no. 3. (July 2014): 1121–1155. doi: 10.1002/cphy.c130054.

Mavropoulos, John C., et al. "The Effects of a Low-Carbohydrate, Ketogenic Diet on the Polycystic Ovary Syndrome: A Pilot Study." *Nutrition & Metabolism* 2, no. 35. (2005). doi: 10.1186/1743-7075-2-35.

McGrice, Melanie, and Judi Porter. "The Effect of Low Carbohydrate Diets on Fertility Hormones and Outcomes in Overweight and Obese Women: A Systematic Review." *Nutrients* 9, no. 3. (March 2017): 204. doi: 10.3390/nu9030204.

Paoli, A., et al. "Beyond Weight Loss: A Review of the Therapeutic Uses of Very-Low-Carbohydrate (Ketogenic) Diets." *European Journal of Clinical Nutrition* 67, no. 8. (August 2013): 789–796. doi: 10.1038/ejcn.2013.116.

Rozing, Maarten P., et al. "Low Serum Free Triiodothyronine Levels Mark Familial Longevity: The Leiden Longevity Study." *The Journals of Gerontology: Series A*, 65A, no. 4 (April 2010): 365–368. doi: 10.1093/gerona/glp200.

Shimazu, Tadahiro, et al. "Suppression of Oxidative Stress by β-Hydroxybutyrate, an Endogenous Histone Deacetylase Inhibitor." *Science* 339, no. 6116. (January 2013): 211–214. doi: 10.1126/science.1227166.

Recipe Index

A

Aioli (Fancy Mayo), 208
Air-Fried Vanilla and Chocolate Layer Cake, 188–189
Almond Meal–Crusted Chicken Fingers, 135–136
Asian Cucumber Salad, 94
Asparagus & Fennel Frittata, 100–101
Asparagus Wrapped in Salmon Bacon, 74
Avocado Brownies, 183
Avocado Fries, 75
Avocado "Toast," 141–142

B

Basic Chicken Salad in Lettuce Cups, 85
Bean-Free Hummus, 211
Beef & Broccoli Pizza, 148–149
Beef Burgers with Bacon, 172–173
Beef Stroganoff, 175–176
Bone Broth, 203–204
Breakfast Bowl with Cauliflower Hash, 59–60
Breakfast Sausage, 58
Brisket Nachos, 155–156
Brussels Sprouts & Ground Beef Scrambled Eggs, 49
Butternut Squash "Cheese" Sauce, 216

C

Cake or Cookie Dough Balls, 193
Cauliflower Mac & Cheese, 113
Cauliflower 'N' Oatmeal, 50
Cauliflower Popcorn, 67
Cauliflower "Potato" Salad, 95
Cauliflower Smoothie, 199
Chicken & Bacon Salad with Sun-Dried Tomato Dressing, 83–84
Chicken Fajitas, 144–145
Chicken Shawarma, 133–134
Chicken Soup, 86
Chicken Teriyaki, 131–132
Chocolate Sandwich Cookies, 184–185
Chopped Bitter Greens Salad, 89
Chorizo Sliders, 160–161
Churros, 191–192
Cobb Salad, 92–93
Coconut Flour–Based Chocolate Chip Waffles, 51
Coffee Cake, 61
Cottage Pie Muffins, 153–154

D

Dairy-Free White Chocolate Bark, 180
Deviled Eggs (7 Variations), 64–66

E

Eggplant Chips, 72–73
Eggplant Dip, 213–214
Eggs Benedict on Grilled Portobello Mushroom Caps, 54–55

F

Fettuccine Alfredo (2 Variations), 111–112
French Toast, 56–57

G

Green Vegetable Stir-Fry with Tofu, 114–115
Grilled Steak with Chimichurri, 157–158
Ground Beef Cauli-Fried Rice, 150–151
Guacamole, 210

H

Halibut Curry, 129–130
Hearts of Palm Linguine with Butternut Squash "Cheese" Sauce, 110
Hot Cocoa/Chocolate Milk, 205

L

Leek & Cauliflower Soup, 82

Lemon–Poppy Seed Muffins, 77

Lobster BLT Salad, 96–97

M

Mayo-Less Tuna Salad, 124

Meatloaf Muffins, 137–138

Meat Waffles/ Bagels, 52–53

Meatza, 152

Mediterranean Spaghetti, 104–105

Mezze Cake, 139–140

Minestrone Soup, 90–91

N

Nachos (3 Variations), 76

Niçoise Salad, 80–81

Nut-Free Pesto, 212

P

Pigs in a Blanket, 68–69

Pork Chops Smothered in Caramelized Onions & Leeks, 177

Pork Pho with Shirataki Noodles, 168–169

Pork Spring Rolls, 164–165

Pork Tacos/Burrito Wraps, 158–159

Pumpkin Pie Smoothie, 196

Pumpkin Spice Latte, 198

R

Roasted Brussels Sprouts & Poached Eggs, 108–109

Roasted Cabbage "Steaks," 103

Roasted Vegetable Salad, 87–88

S

Salmon Poke, 118

Salmon with Mustard Sauce, 120–121

Sautéed Asparagus with Beef Jerky Sticks, 70

Scampi Sauce, 215

Scotch Eggs, 71

Sesame-Crusted Tuna, 119

Shakshuka, 102

Simple Ice Cream with 8 Flavor Customizations, 181–182

Simply Broiled or Air-Fried Salmon, 125

Slow-Cooked Shredded Beef, 174–175

Snickerdoodle Pudding, 190

Spaghetti Squash & Ground Pork Stir-Fry with Kale, 170–171

Spaghetti Squash Puttanesca, 122–123

Stuffed Bell Peppers, 166–167

Stuffed Eggplant, 106–107

Sushi, 127–128

Sweet Egg Salad, 186–187

T

Tandoori Beef Fajitas, 162–163

Turkey-Stuffed Avocados, 143

V

Vanilla and/or Chocolate Dipping Sauce, 209

Virgin (or Not) Bloody Mary, 200–201

Virgin (or Not) Eggnog, 197

Virgin (or Not) Mojito, 202

W

Whole Roasted Sea Bass, 126

Winter Squash Pancakes, 48

Y

Yum Yum Sauce, 217

Index

A

Adenosine, 11

Almond milk
  Cauliflower
    Smoothie, 199
  French Toast, 56–57

Anchovies
  Niçoise Salad, 80–81
  Pork Pho with
    Shirataki Noo-
    dles, 168–169
  Spaghetti Squash
    Puttanesca,
    122–123

Artichoke hearts
  Mediterranean Spa-
    ghetti, 104–105
  Mezze Cake, 139–140
  Spaghetti Squash Put-
    tanesca, 122–123

Arugula
  Chopped Bitter
    Greens Salad, 89

Asparagus
  Asparagus & Fennel
    Frittata, 100–101
  Asparagus Wrapped in
    Salmon Bacon, 74
  Ground Beef
    Cauli-Fried
    Rice, 150–151
  Nut-Free Pesto, 212
  Roasted Vegetable
    Salad, 87–88

Sautéed Asparagus
    with Beef Jerky
    Sticks, 70
  Stuffed Egg-
    plant, 106–107
  Tandoori Beef Faji-
    tas, 162–163
  Turkey-Stuffed Avo-
    cados, 143

Autoimmune condi-
  tions, 12

Avocados
  Avocado
    Brownies, 183
  Avocado Fries, 75
  Avocado
    "Toast," 141–142
  Chicken & Bacon
    Salad with
    Sun-Dried Tomato
    Dressing, 83–84
  Cobb Salad, 92–93
  Deviled Eggs
    (7 Variations),
    64–66
  Green Vegetable
    Stir-Fry with
    Tofu, 114–115
  Guacamole, 210
  Lobster BLT
    Salad, 96–97
  Snickerdoodle Pud-
    ding, 190
  Sushi, 127–128

Turkey-Stuffed Avo-
    cados, 143
  Vanilla and/or Choco-
    late Dipping
    Sauce, 209

B

Bacon
  Beef Burgers with
    Bacon, 172–173
  Chicken & Bacon
    Salad with
    Sun-Dried Tomato
    Dressing, 83–84
  Cobb Salad, 92–93
  Eggs Benedict on
    Grilled Portobello
    Mushroom
    Caps, 54–55
  Lobster BLT
    Salad, 96–97

Basil
  Mediterranean Spa-
    ghetti, 104–105
  Nut-Free Pesto, 212
  Stuffed Bell Pep-
    pers, 166–167
  Stuffed Egg-
    plant, 106–107

Beef
  Beef & Broccoli
    Pizza, 148–149
  Beef Burgers with
    Bacon, 172–173

Beef *(Continued)*
  Beef Stroganoff,
    175–176
  Breakfast Sausage, 58
  Brisket
    Nachos, 155–156
  Brussels Sprouts &
    Ground Beef
    Scrambled Eggs, 49
  Deviled Eggs
    (7 Variations),
    64–66
  Grilled Steak with
    Chimichurri,
    157–158
  Ground Beef
    Cauli-Fried
    Rice, 150–151
  Meat Waffles/
    Bagels, 52–53
  Meatza, 152
  Pigs in a Blan-
    ket, 68–69
  Sautéed Asparagus
    with Beef Jerky
    Sticks, 70
  Scotch Eggs, 71
  Slow-Cooked Shred-
    ded Beef, 174–175
  Stuffed Bell Pep-
    pers, 166–167
  Tandoori Beef
    Fajitas, 162–163
Beverages. See
  also Smoothies
  Bone Broth, 203–204
  Hot Cocoa/Chocolate
    Milk, 205
  Pumpkin Spice
    Latte, 198
  Virgin (or Not) Bloody
    Mary, 200–201

Virgin (or Not)
    Eggnog, 197
  Virgin (or Not)
    Mojito, 202
Bison
  Breakfast Sausage, 58
  Grilled Steak with
    Chimichurri,
    157–158
  Meat Waffles/
    Bagels, 52–53
Broccoli
  Beef & Broccoli
    Pizza, 148–149
Brussels sprouts
  Brussels Sprouts &
    Ground Beef
    Scrambled Eggs, 49
  Deviled Eggs
    (7 Variations),
    64–66
  Green Vegetable
    Stir-Fry with
    Tofu, 114–115
  Minestrone
    Soup, 90–91
  Roasted Brussels
    Sprouts & Poached
    Eggs, 108–109
  Roasted Vegetable
    Salad, 87–88
Bulk cooking, 22
Bulk Cook recipes
  Aioli (Fancy
    Mayo), 208
  Almond Meal–Crusted
    Chicken Fingers,
    135–136
  Asparagus & Fennel
    Frittata, 100–101
  Asparagus Wrapped in
    Salmon Bacon, 74

Avocado
    Brownies, 183
Bean-Free
    Hummus, 211
Beef Stroga-
    noff, 175–176
Breakfast Sausage, 58
Butternut Squash
    "Cheese"
    Sauce, 216
Cake or Cookie Dough
    Balls, 193
Cauliflower Mac
    & Cheese, 113
Cauliflower
    Popcorn, 67
Cauliflower "Potato"
    Salad, 95
Chicken Faji-
    tas, 144–145
Chicken Sha-
    warma, 133–134
Chicken Soup, 86
Chicken Teriyaki,
    131–132
Chocolate
    Sandwich
    Cookies, 184–185
Chorizo Sliders,
    160–161
Cottage Pie Muffins,
    153–154
Dairy-Free White
    Chocolate
    Bark, 180
Eggplant
    Chips, 72–73
Eggplant
    Dip, 213–214
Grilled Steak with
    Chimichurri,
    157–158

Ground Beef
Cauli-Fried
Rice, 150–151
Halibut
Curry, 129–130
Lemon–Poppy Seed
Muffins, 77
Mayo-Less Tuna
Salad, 124
Meatloaf Muf-
fins, 137–138
Mezze Cake,
139–140
Minestrone
Soup, 90–91
Nut-Free Pesto, 212
Pork Chops Smothered
in Caramelized
Onions &
Leeks, 177
Scampi Sauce, 215
Shakshuka, 102
Slow-Cooked
Shredded
Beef, 174–175
Snickerdoodle
Pudding, 190
Spaghetti Squash &
Ground Pork
Stir-Fry with
Kale, 170–171
Tandoori Beef Fajitas,
162–163
Yum Yum Sauce, 217
B Vitamins, 5

C
Cabbage
Beef Burgers with
Bacon, 172–173
Chopped Bitter
Greens Salad, 89
Green Vegetable
Stir-Fry with
Tofu, 114–115
Roasted Cabbage
"Steaks," 103
Calcium, 5
Calories, 6, 14
Capers
Mediterranean Spa-
ghetti, 104–105
Niçoise Salad, 80–81
Salmon Poke, 118
Spaghetti Squash
Puttanesca,
122–123
Carbohydrates, 4, 6–8, 14
Carrots
Cottage Pie Muf-
fins, 153–154
Meatloaf Muf-
fins, 137–138
Meatza, 152
Minestrone
Soup, 90–91
Pork Spring
Rolls, 164–165
Cauliflower
Breakfast Bowl with
Cauliflower
Hash, 59–60
Cauliflower Mac &
Cheese, 113
Cauliflower
'N' Oatmeal, 50
Cauliflower
Popcorn, 67
Cauliflower "Potato"
Salad, 95
Cauliflower
Smoothie, 199
Cottage Pie Muf-
fins, 153–154
Leek & Cauliflower
Soup, 82
Cauliflower rice
Chicken Sha-
warma, 133–134
Chicken Teri-
yaki, 131–132
French Toast, 56–57
Ground Beef
Cauli-Fried
Rice, 150–151
Halibut
Curry, 129–130
Meatza, 152
Mezze Cake, 139–140
Sushi, 127–128
Celery
Basic Chicken Salad
in Lettuce
Cups, 85
Bone Broth, 203–204
Cauliflower "Potato"
Salad, 95
Cottage Pie Muf-
fins, 153–154
Halibut
Curry, 129–130
Minestrone
Soup, 90–91
Celery root
Brisket
Nachos, 155–156
Cheese
Asparagus & Fennel
Frittata, 100–101
Beef & Broccoli
Pizza, 148–149
Beef Burgers with
Bacon, 172–173
Breakfast Bowl with
Cauliflower
Hash, 59–60

Cheese (Continued)
  Chorizo Slid-
    ers, 160–161
  Cobb Salad, 92–93
  Cottage Pie Muf-
    fins, 153–154
  Fettuccine Alfredo
    (2 Variations),
    111–112
  Meatza, 152
  Mediterranean
    Spaghetti,
    104–105
  Nachos
    (3 Variations), 76
  Roasted Vegetable
    Salad, 87–88
  Shakshuka, 102
  Spaghetti Squash Put-
    tanesca, 122–123
  Stuffed Bell Pep-
    pers, 166–167
  Stuffed Egg-
    plant, 106–107
Chicken
  Almond Meal–Crusted
    Chicken Fingers,
    135–136
  Basic Chicken Salad in
    Lettuce Cups, 85
  Breakfast Sausage, 58
  Chicken & Bacon
    Salad with
    Sun-Dried Tomato
    Dressing, 83–84
  Chicken Faji-
    tas, 144–145
  Chicken Sha-
    warma, 133–134
  Chicken Soup, 86

Chicken Teri-
  yaki, 131–132
Deviled Eggs
  (7 Variations),
  64–66
Mezze Cake, 139–140
Pigs in a Blan-
  ket, 68–69
Chives
  Cauliflower "Potato"
    Salad, 95
  Lobster BLT
    Salad, 96–97
Chocolate. See also
  White chocolate
  Air-Fried Vanilla and
    Chocolate Layer
    Cake, 188–189
  Avocado
    Brownies, 183
  Cake or Cookie Dough
    Balls, 193
  Cauliflower
    Smoothie, 199
  Chocolate Sandwich
    Cookies, 184–185
  Coconut Flour–Based
    Chocolate Chip
    Waffles, 51
  Hot Cocoa/Chocolate
    Milk, 205
  Simple Ice Cream
    with 8 Flavor
    Customizations,
    181–182
  Sweet Egg
    Salad, 186–187
  Vanilla and/or Choco-
    late Dipping
    Sauce, 209

Cilantro
  Chopped Bitter
    Greens Salad, 89
  Guacamole, 210
  Pork Pho with
    Shirataki
    Noodles, 168–169
  Pork Tacos/Burrito
    Wraps, 158–159
  Shakshuka, 102
Coconut
  Simple Ice Cream with
    8 Flavor Customi-
    zations, 181–182
Coconut cream
  Fettuccine Alfredo
    (2 Variations),
    111–112
  Pumpkin Pie
    Smoothie,
    196
Coconut milk
  Air-Fried Vanilla and
    Chocolate Layer
    Cake, 188–189
  Asparagus & Fennel
    Frittata, 100–101
  Avocado
    Brownies, 183
  Cauliflower
    Smoothie, 199
  Chocolate Sandwich
    Cookies, 184–185
  Churros, 191–192
  Cottage Pie Muf-
    fins, 153–154
  Dairy-Free White
    Chocolate
    Bark, 180
  French Toast, 56–57

Halibut
Curry, 129–130
Hot Cocoa/Chocolate
Milk, 205
Simple Ice Cream with
8 Flavor Customi-
zations, 181–182
Sweet Egg
Salad, 186–187
Vanilla and/or Choco-
late Dipping
Sauce, 209
Virgin (or Not)
Eggnog, 197
Coffee
Coffee Cake, 61
Pumpkin Spice
Latte, 198
Cortisol, 13
Cucumbers
Asian Cucumber
Salad, 94
Salmon Poke, 118
Sushi, 127–128

D
Dandelion greens
Chopped Bitter
Greens Salad, 89
Desserts
Air-Fried Vanilla and
Chocolate Layer
Cake, 188–189
Avocado
Brownies, 183
Cake or Cookie Dough
Balls, 193
Chocolate Sandwich
Cookies, 184–185
Churros, 191–192

Dairy-Free White
Chocolate
Bark, 180
Simple Ice Cream
with 8 Flavor
Customiza-
tions, 181–182
Snickerdoodle Pud-
ding, 190
Sweet Egg
Salad, 186–187
Dill
Basic Chicken Salad in
Lettuce Cups, 85
Cottage Pie Muf-
fins, 153–154
Dips
Aioli (Fancy
Mayo), 208
Bean-Free
Hummus, 211
Guacamole, 210
Vanilla and/or
Chocolate Dipping
Sauce, 209

E
Eggplant
Eggplant
Chips, 72–73
Eggplant
Dip, 213–214
Meatza, 152
Mediterranean Spa-
ghetti, 104–105
Mezze Cake, 139–140
Nachos
(3 Variations), 76
Pigs in a Blan-
ket, 68–69

Roasted Vegetable
Salad, 87–88
Stuffed Egg-
plant, 106–107
Eggs
Aioli (Fancy
Mayo), 208
Air-Fried Vanilla and
Chocolate Layer
Cake, 188–189
Almond Meal–Crusted
Chicken Fin-
gers, 135–136
Asparagus & Fennel
Frittata, 100–101
Avocado
Brownies, 183
Avocado Fries, 75
Beef Burgers with
Bacon, 172–173
Brussels Sprouts
& Ground
Beef Scrambled
Eggs, 49
Cauliflower "Potato"
Salad, 95
Churros, 191–192
Cobb Salad, 92–93
Coffee Cake, 61
Deviled Eggs
(7 Variations),
64–66
Eggs Benedict on
Grilled Portobello
Mushroom
Caps, 54–55
French Toast, 56–57
Ground Beef
Cauli-Fried
Rice, 150–151

Eggs *(Continued)*
    Lemon–Poppy Seed
        Muffins, 77
    Meatloaf Muf-
        fins, 137–138
    Meat Waffles/
        Bagels, 52–53
    Niçoise Salad,
        80–81
    Pork Spring
        Rolls, 164–165
    Roasted Brussels
        Sprouts &
        Poached Eggs,
        108–109
    Sautéed Asparagus
        with Beef Jerky
        Sticks, 70
    Scampi Sauce, 215
    Scotch Eggs, 71
    Shakshuka, 102
    Stuffed Egg-
        plant, 106–107
    Sweet Egg
        Salad, 186–187
    Winter Squash
        Pancakes, 48
Endive
    Chopped Bitter
        Greens Salad, 89
Endometriosis, 12
Energy, 10
Erythritol, 24
Estrogen dominance, 13
Exercise, 15

F

Fasting, 9
Fat metabolism, 13
Fats, 6–8, 15, 18
Female, use of term, 4

Fennel
    Asparagus & Fennel
        Frittata, 100–101
    Roasted Vegetable
        Salad, 87–88
Fish
    Asian Cucumber
        Salad, 94
    Asparagus Wrapped in
        Salmon Bacon, 74
    Deviled Eggs
        (7 Variations),
        64–66
    Halibut
        Curry, 129–130
    Mayo-Less Tuna
        Salad, 124
    Niçoise Salad, 80–81
    Salmon Poke, 118
    Salmon with Mustard
        Sauce, 120–121
    Sesame-Crusted
        Tuna, 119
    Simply Broiled or
        Air-Fried
        Salmon, 125
    Spaghetti Squash Put-
        tanesca, 122–123
    Sushi, 127–128
    Whole Roasted Sea
        Bass, 126
Flax milk
    Cauliflower
        'N' Oatmeal, 50
    Pumpkin Spice
        Latte, 198

G

Ginger
    Asian Cucumber
        Salad, 94

Ground Beef
    Cauli-Fried
        Rice, 150–151
    Pork Pho with
        Shirataki Noodles,
        168–169
    Pork Spring
        Rolls, 164–165
Gluconeogenesis, 7
Glucose, 6–7, 8, 13
Glycogen, 7
Green beans
    Minestrone
        Soup, 90–91
    Niçoise Salad, 80–81
Greens. See also specific
    Chicken Shawarma,
        133–134
    Roasted Vegetable
        Salad, 87–88

H

Hearts of palm
    Fettuccine Alfredo
        (2 Variations),
        111–112
    Hearts of Palm
        Linguine with
        Butternut Squash
        "Cheese"
        Sauce, 110
    Mediterranean
        Spaghetti,
        104–105
Hemp milk
    Pumpkin Pie
        Smoothie, 196
Hofmekler, Ori, 9
Hormones, 13
HPA axis dysfunction, 13

I

Ice cream
    Coconut Flour–Based
        Chocolate Chip
        Waffles, 51
    Simple Ice Cream with
        8 Flavor Customi-
        zations, 181–182
Inflammation, 11
Ingredients
    pantry, 24
    perishable, 23–24
    special, 25–26
Insulin, 7, 13
Intermittent fasting, 9
Intuitive eating, 43
Iodine, 5
Iron, 5

J

Jicama
    Basic Chicken Salad in
        Lettuce Cups, 85
    Cobb Salad, 92–93
    Mayo-Less Tuna
        Salad, 124
    Pork Spring
        Rolls, 164–165

K

Kale
    Green Vegetable
        Stir-Fry with
        Tofu, 114–115
    Minestrone
        Soup, 90–91
    Spaghetti Squash &
        Ground Pork
        Stir-Fry with
        Kale, 170–171

Keto brands, 25–26
Keto flu, 21
Ketogenic diet
    about, 4, 6
    benefits of, 10–13
    and the female
        body, 13
    foods to avoid, 19
    foods to
        embrace, 18–19
    how it works, 6–8
    tips, 14–15, 43
Ketones, 8
Ketosis, 7
Kohlrabi
    Niçoise Salad, 80–81

L

Leeks
    Green Vegetable
        Stir-Fry with
        Tofu, 114–115
    Leek & Cauliflower
        Soup, 82
    Pork Chops Smothered
        in Caramelized
        Onions &
        Leeks, 177
    Whole Roasted Sea
        Bass, 126
Leftovers, 22–23
Lemongrass
    Pork Pho with
        Shirataki
        Noodles, 168–169
Lemons
    Aioli (Fancy
        Mayo), 208
    Basic Chicken Salad in
        Lettuce Cups, 85

Bean-Free
    Hummus, 211
Beef Stroga-
    noff, 175–176
Chicken & Bacon
    Salad with
    Sun-Dried Tomato
    Dressing, 83–84
Chicken Teri-
    yaki, 131–132
Eggplant
    Dip, 213–214
Eggs Benedict on
    Grilled Portobello
    Mushroom
    Caps, 54–55
Lemon–Poppy Seed
    Muffins, 77
Nut-Free Pesto, 212
Salmon Poke, 118
Salmon with Mustard
    Sauce, 120–121
Scampi Sauce, 215
Virgin (or Not)
    Bloody
    Mary, 200–201
Whole Roasted Sea
    Bass, 126
Lettuce
    Basic Chicken Salad in
        Lettuce Cups, 85
    Chicken & Bacon
        Salad with
        Sun-Dried Tomato
        Dressing, 83–84
    Chicken Faji-
        tas, 144–145
    Chorizo Slid-
        ers, 160–161
    Cobb Salad, 92–93

Lettuce (Continued)
  Lobster BLT
    Salad, 96–97
  Niçoise Salad, 80–81
  Pork Tacos/Burrito
    Wraps, 158–159
  Tandoori Beef Faji-
    tas, 162–163
Limes
  Avocado
    "Toast," 141–142
  Guacamole, 210
  Pork Pho with
    Shirataki Noo-
    dles, 168–169
  Virgin (or Not)
    Mojito, 202
Lobsters
  Lobster BLT
    Salad, 96–97

M
Macronutrients, 7–8, 20.
    See also Carbohy-
    drates; Fats; Proteins
Magnesium, 5
Meal planning
  21-day plan notes, 27
  about, 20, 22–23
  building your own
    plan, 42
  week one, 28–32
  week three, 37–41
  week two, 33–36
Meat bones. See also
    specific meats
  Bone Broth, 203–204
Mental clarity, 10
Micronutrients, 4–6
Mint
  Virgin (or Not)
    Mojito, 202

Mushrooms
  Asparagus & Fennel
    Frittata, 100–101
  Beef Stroga-
    noff, 175–176
  Chorizo Slid-
    ers, 160–161
  Cottage Pie Muf-
    fins, 153–154
  Eggs Benedict on
    Grilled Portobello
    Mushroom
    Caps, 54–55
  Meatloaf Muf-
    fins, 137–138
  Tandoori Beef Faji-
    tas, 162–163

N
Nutritional needs, 4–6
Nuts
  Basic Chicken Salad
    in Lettuce
    Cups, 85
  Cake or Cookie Dough
    Balls, 193
  Simple Ice Cream with
    8 Flavor Customi-
    zations, 181–182

O
Olives
  Beef & Broccoli
    Pizza, 148–149
  Eggplant
    Dip, 213–214
  Mayo-Less Tuna
    Salad, 124
  Mediterranean
    Spaghetti,
    104–105
  Mezze Cake, 139–140

Niçoise Salad, 80–81
  Spaghetti Squash
    Puttanesca,
    122–123
One pot/pan recipes
  Asparagus Wrapped in
    Salmon Bacon, 74
  Beef Stroga-
    noff, 175–176
  Bone Broth, 203–204
  Breakfast Sausage, 58
  Cauliflower
    Popcorn, 67
  Chicken Soup, 86
  Fettuccine Alfredo
    (2 Variations),
    111–112
  Green Vegetable
    Stir-Fry with
    Tofu, 114–115
  Ground Beef
    Cauli-Fried
    Rice, 150–151
  Halibut
    Curry, 129–130
  Hearts of Palm
    Linguine with
    Butternut Squash
    "Cheese"
    Sauce, 110
  Mediterranean
    Spaghetti,
    104–105
  Mezze Cake, 139–140
  Minestrone
    Soup, 90–91
  Pigs in a Blan-
    ket, 68–69
  Pumpkin Spice
    Latte, 198
  Roasted Cabbage
    "Steaks," 103

Salmon Poke, 118
Sautéed Asparagus
    with Beef Jerky
    Sticks, 70
Shakshuka, 102
Simply Broiled or
    Air-Fried
    Salmon, 125
Slow-Cooked
    Shredded
    Beef, 174–175
Spaghetti Squash
    & Ground Pork
    Stir-Fry with
    Kale, 170–171
Whole Roasted Sea
    Bass, 126

P
Pantry staples, 24
Parsley
    Basic Chicken Salad
        in Lettuce
        Cups, 85
    Beef Stroganoff,
        175–176
    Bone Broth,
        203–204
    Breakfast Sausage, 58
    Cauliflower Mac &
        Cheese, 113
    Chopped Bitter
        Greens Salad, 89
    Eggplant
        Dip, 213–214
    Eggs Benedict on
        Grilled Portobello
        Mushroom
        Caps, 54–55
    Grilled Steak with
        Chimichurri,
        157–158

Hearts of Palm Lin-
    guine with
    Butternut Squash
    "Cheese"
    Sauce, 110
Leek & Cauliflower
    Soup, 82
Mediterranean Spa-
    ghetti, 104–105
Scampi Sauce, 215
Spaghetti Squash
    Puttanesca,
    122–123
Stuffed Egg-
    plant, 106–107
Peppers, bell
    Basic Chicken
        Salad in Lettuce
        Cups, 85
    Chicken Faji-
        tas, 144–145
    Meatloaf Muf-
        fins, 137–138
    Shakshuka, 102
    Stuffed Bell Pep-
        pers, 166–167
    Stuffed Egg-
        plant, 106–107
    Tandoori Beef Faji-
        tas, 162–163
Peppers, jalapeño
    Guacamole, 210
Polycystic ovary syn-
    drome (PCOS), 11–12
Pork. See also Bacon
    Breakfast Sausage, 58
    Chorizo Slid-
        ers, 160–161
    Cottage Pie Muf-
        fins, 153–154
    Meat Waffles/
        Bagels, 52–53

Pork Chops Smothered
    in Caramelized
    Onions &
    Leeks, 177
Pork Pho with Shirataki
    Noodles, 168–169
Pork Spring
    Rolls, 164–165
Pork Tacos/Burrito
    Wraps, 158–159
Spaghetti Squash &
    Ground Pork
    Stir-Fry with
    Kale, 170–171
Stuffed Bell Pep-
    pers, 166–167
Proteins, 7–8, 14, 18
Pumpkin
    Pumpkin Pie
        Smoothie, 196
    Roasted Vegetable
        Salad, 87–88

R
Radicchio
    Chopped Bitter
        Greens Salad, 89
Refrigerator staples, 23–24
Rosemary
    Scampi Sauce, 215
Rutabagas
    Brisket
        Nachos, 155–156
    Leek & Cauliflower
        Soup, 82

S
Salads
    Asian Cucumber
        Salad, 94
    Basic Chicken
        Salad in Lettuce
        Cups, 85

Salads *(Continued)*
  Chicken & Bacon Salad
    with Sun-Dried
    Tomato Dress-
    ing, 83–84
  Chopped Bitter
    Greens Salad, 89
  Cobb Salad, 92–93
  Mayo-Less Tuna
    Salad, 124
  Niçoise Salad, 80–81
  Roasted Vegetable
    Salad, 87–88
  Sweet Egg
    Salad, 186–187
Salmon
  Asian Cucumber
    Salad, 94
  Asparagus Wrapped in
    Salmon Bacon, 74
  Deviled Eggs
    (7 Variations),
    64–66
  Salmon Poke, 118
  Salmon with Mustard
    Sauce, 120–121
  Simply Broiled or
    Air-Fried
    Salmon, 125
Sardines
  Deviled Eggs
    (7 Variations),
    64–66
Sauces
  Aioli (Fancy
    Mayo), 208
  Butternut Squash
    "Cheese"
    Sauce, 216
  Nut-Free Pesto, 212
  Scampi Sauce, 215

  Vanilla and/or Choco-
    late Dipping
    Sauce, 209
  Yum Yum
    Sauce, 217
Sausage
  Beef & Broccoli
    Pizza, 148–149
  Breakfast Bowl with
    Cauliflower
    Hash, 59–60
  Breakfast Sausage, 58
  Chorizo Slid-
    ers, 160–161
  Mezze Cake, 139–140
Self-kindness, 43
Shirataki noodles
  Beef Stroganoff,
    175–176
  Fettuccine Alfredo
    (2 Variations),
    111–112
  Pork Pho with
    Shirataki Noo-
    dles, 168–169
Skin, 11
Sleep, 11
Smoothies
  Cauliflower
    Smoothie, 199
  Pumpkin Pie
    Smoothie, 196
Snacks, 27
Soups
  Chicken Soup, 86
  Leek & Cauliflower
    Soup, 82
  Minestrone
    Soup, 90–91
  Pork Pho with Shirataki
    Noodles, 168–169

Spinach
  Almond Meal–Crusted
    Chicken Fin-
    gers, 135–136
  Breakfast Bowl with
    Cauliflower
    Hash, 59–60
  Brisket
    Nachos, 155–156
  Chicken Soup, 86
  Eggs Benedict on
    Grilled Portobello
    Mushroom
    Caps, 54–55
  Green Vegetable
    Stir-Fry with
    Tofu, 114–115
  Mayo-Less Tuna
    Salad, 124
  Pork Spring
    Rolls, 164–165
  Turkey-Stuffed Avo-
    cados, 143
Squash. See also
    Zucchini
  Butternut Squash
    "Cheese"
    Sauce, 216
  Cauliflower Mac &
    Cheese, 113
  Cauliflower
    Smoothie, 199
  Deviled Eggs
    (7 Variations),
    64–66
  Fettuccine Alfredo
    (2 Variations),
    111–112
  Halibut
    Curry, 129–130

Hearts of Palm
 Linguine with
 Butternut Squash
 "Cheese"
 Sauce, 110
Mediterranean Spa-
 ghetti, 104–105
Nachos
 (3 Variations), 76
Pork Spring
 Rolls, 164–165
Spaghetti Squash &
 Ground Pork
 Stir-Fry with
 Kale, 170–171
Spaghetti Squash
 Puttanesca,
 122–123
Winter Squash Pan-
 cakes, 48
Stress, 43
Super Quick recipes, 215
 Aioli (Fancy
 Mayo), 208
 Almond Meal–Crusted
 Chicken Fin-
 gers, 135–136
 Asian Cucumber
 Salad, 94
 Avocado Fries, 75
 Avocado
 "Toast," 141–142
 Basic Chicken Salad in
 Lettuce Cups, 85
 Bean-Free
 Hummus, 211
 Breakfast Bowl with
 Cauliflower
 Hash, 59–60

Breakfast Sausage, 58
Brussels Sprouts &
 Ground Beef
 Scrambled Eggs, 49
Butternut Squash
 "Cheese"
 Sauce, 216
Cauliflower Mac &
 Cheese, 113
Cauliflower
 'N' Oatmeal, 50
Cauliflower "Potato"
 Salad, 95
Cauliflower
 Smoothie, 199
Chicken & Bacon
 Salad with
 Sun-Dried
 Tomato Dress-
 ing, 83–84
Chicken Faji-
 tas, 144–145
Chopped Bitter
 Greens Salad, 89
Cobb Salad, 92–93
Coconut Flour–Based
 Chocolate Chip
 Waffles, 51
Deviled Eggs
 (7 Variations),
 64–66
Eggs Benedict on
 Grilled Portobello
 Mushroom
 Caps, 54–55
Fettuccine Alfredo
 (2 Variations),
 111–112

Green Vegetable
 Stir-Fry with
 Tofu, 114–115
Grilled Steak with
 Chimichurri,
 157–158
Ground Beef
 Cauli-Fried
 Rice, 150–151
Hearts of Palm Lin-
 guine with
 Butternut Squash
 "Cheese"
 Sauce, 110
Hot Cocoa/Chocolate
 Milk, 205
Lobster BLT
 Salad, 96–97
Mayo-Less Tuna
 Salad, 124
Meat Waffles/
 Bagels, 52–53
Mediterranean Spa-
 ghetti, 104–105
Nut-Free Pesto, 212
Pigs in a Blan-
 ket, 68–69
Pork Chops Smothered
 in Caramelized
 Onions &
 Leeks, 177
Pumpkin Pie
 Smoothie, 196
Pumpkin Spice
 Latte, 198
Salmon Poke, 118
Sautéed Asparagus
 with Beef Jerky
 Sticks, 70

Super Quick recipes
    (Continued)
    Sesame-Crusted
        Tuna, 119
    Snickerdoodle Pud-
        ding, 190
    Sushi, 127–128
    Sweet Egg
        Salad, 186–187
    Turkey-Stuffed Avo-
        cados, 143
    Vanilla and/or Choco-
        late Dipping
        Sauce, 209
    Virgin (or Not)
        Bloody Mary,
        200–201
    Virgin (or Not)
        Eggnog, 197
    Virgin (or Not)
        Mojito, 202
    Winter Squash Pan-
        cakes, 48
    Yum Yum Sauce, 217
Sweeteners, 24

T
Thyroid conditions, 13
Tofu
    Green Vegetable
        Stir-Fry with
        Tofu, 114–115
    Stuffed Egg-
        plant, 106–107
Tomatoes
    Asparagus & Fennel
        Frittata, 100–101

Avocado
    "Toast," 141–142
    Beef Burgers with
        Bacon, 172–173
    Chicken & Bacon
        Salad with
        Sun-Dried
        Tomato Dress-
        ing, 83–84
    Chorizo Slid-
        ers, 160–161
    Cobb Salad, 92–93
    Deviled Eggs
        (7 Variations),
        64–66
    Guacamole, 210
    Lobster BLT
        Salad, 96–97
    Minestrone
        Soup, 90–91
    Niçoise Salad, 80–81
    Shakshuka, 102
    Stuffed Egg-
        plant, 106–107
Tomatoes, sun-dried
    Chicken & Bacon
        Salad with
        Sun-Dried
        Tomato Dress-
        ing, 83–84
    Guacamole, 210
    Mayo-Less Tuna
        Salad, 124
    Mezze Cake, 139–140
Tuna
    Asian Cucumber
        Salad, 94

Deviled Eggs
    (7 Variations),
    64–66
Mayo-Less Tuna
    Salad, 124
Niçoise Salad,
    80–81
Sesame-Crusted
    Tuna, 119
Spaghetti Squash
    Puttanesca,
    122–123
Turkey
    Avocado
        "Toast," 141–142
    Breakfast Sausage, 58
    Cobb Salad, 92–93
    Deviled Eggs
        (7 Variations),
        64–66
    Meatloaf Muf-
        fins, 137–138
    Meat Waffles/
        Bagels, 52–53
    Turkey-Stuffed Avo-
        cados, 143

U
Uterine fibroids, 12

V
Vegetables, 18–19. See
    also specific
    Bean-Free
        Hummus, 211
Vitamin D, 5
Volek, Jeff, 12

W

Warrior Diet, 9
Weight loss, 10
White chocolate
    Dairy-Free White
        Chocolate
        Bark, 180
Woman, use of term, 4

Y

Yogurt, coconut
    Air-Fried Vanilla and
        Chocolate Layer
        Cake, 188–189

Beef Stroganoff,
    175–176
Coconut Flour–Based
    Chocolate Chip
    Waffles, 51
Pumpkin Pie
    Smoothie, 196
Yogurt, Greek
    Beef Stroganoff,
        175–176
    Eggplant
        Dip, 213–214
    Tandoori Beef
        Fajitas, 162–163

Z

Zucchini
    Meatza, 152
    Mezze Cake, 139–140
    Roasted Vegetable
        Salad, 87–88

Acknowledgments

First, I'd like to thank my mother for inspiring me to write this book. She is my mentor, my teacher, and my confidante. Mom, without you and your guidance, I would probably still be eating those Brown Sugar Cinnamon Pop-Tarts®, which certainly don't aid in getting into ketosis! This book also wouldn't have been possible because you were eating a keto diet before it ever became popular!

I had my sister-in-law, Ali Stewart, in mind when creating and writing a plethora of the recipes for this book because I've been so inspired by her journey to eat more healthily over the last few years. #MrAirFryer.

I'd also like to thank all of my social media friends for repeatedly telling me to write a book. I'd particularly like to thank Brittany Wilson, who I met through my blog. She motivated me to write this book because I have observed her transformation over the years, confirming that what we eat truly affects all aspects of our lives.

Callisto Media and Pippa White, thank you for your careful edits and passion for eating good food. Our relationship has been a match made in heaven, and I'm so grateful for you.

And I can't forget to thank the flaky reddish-pink fish striped with sexy omega-3-rich marbling that was my brain fuel to write this book. Salmon, thank you for never getting sick of me, because I never, ever get sick of eating you.

CPSIA information can be obtained
at www.ICGtesting.com
Printed in the USA
BVHW062255170519
548220BV00003BD/5/P

9 781641 523578